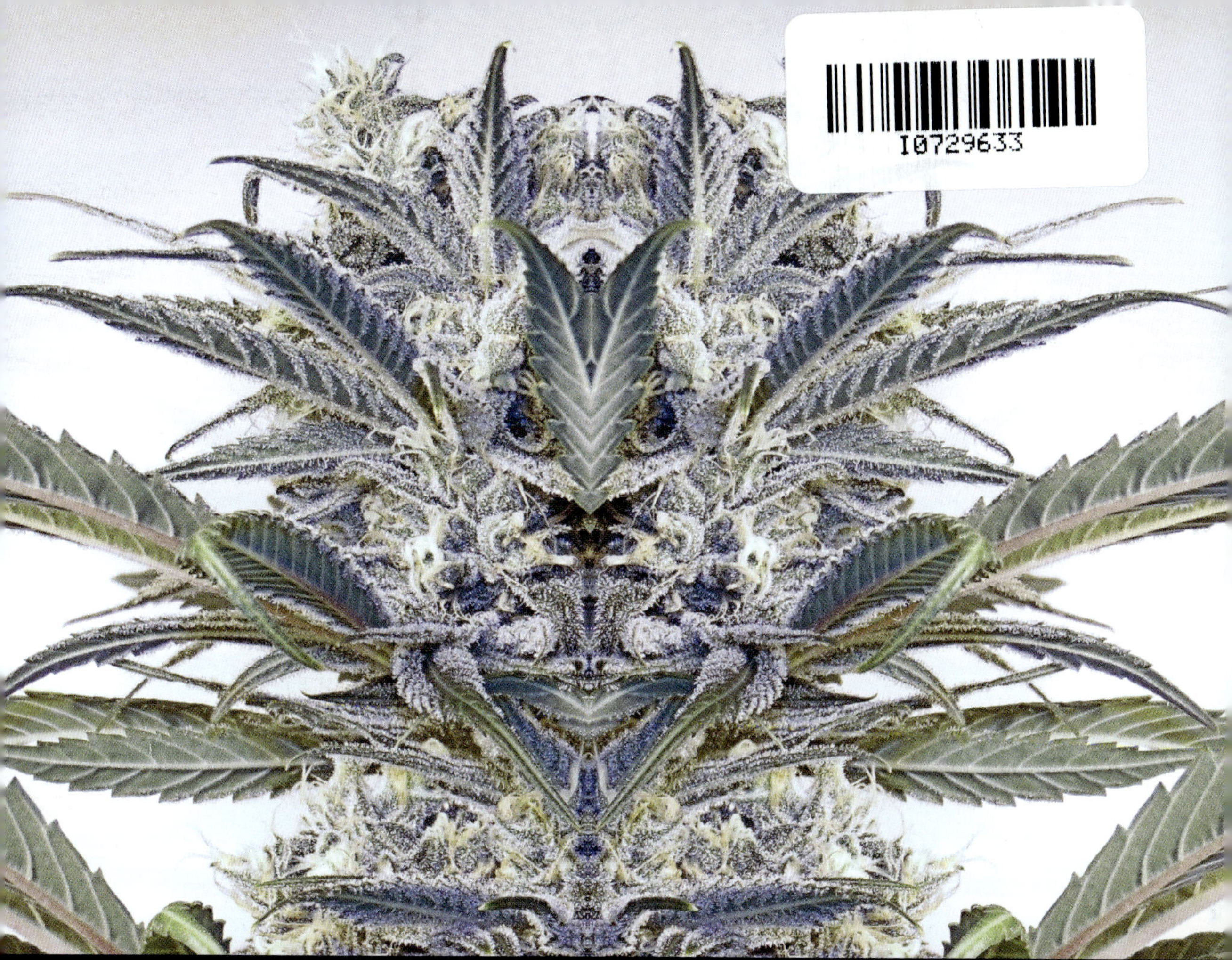

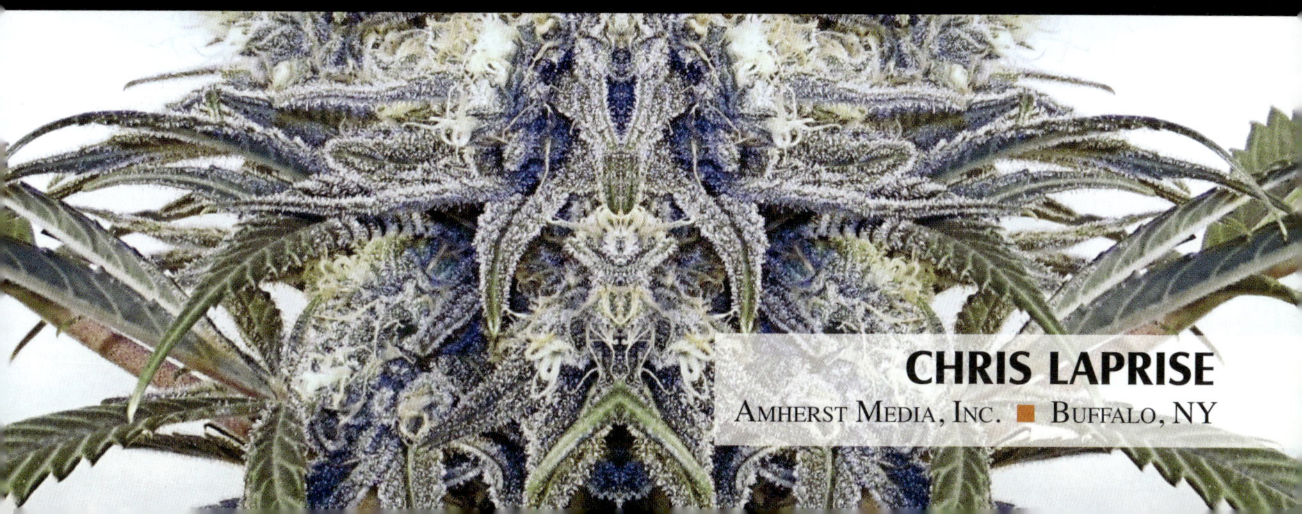

The Art of
Cannabis

A VISUAL TOUR

CHRIS LAPRISE

Amherst Media, Inc. ■ Buffalo, NY

Published by:
Amherst Media, Inc.
PO Box 538
Buffalo, NY 14213
www.AmherstMedia.com

ISBN-13: 978-1-68203-400-2
Library of Congress Control Number: 2018960518
Printed in the United States of America
10 9 8 7 6 5 4 3 2 1

Notice of Disclaimer: The information contained in this book is based on the author's experience and opinions. The author and publisher will not be held liable for the use or misuse of the information in this book.

The information contained in this book is presented for educational purposes only. Check with your local, state, and federal laws regarding possession, consumption, and cultivation of cannabis. If you seek to use cannabis to treat a medical condition, consult with your physician or a licensed health-care provider first.

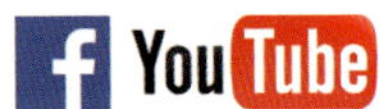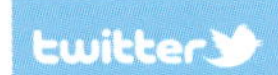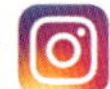

www.facebook.com/AmherstMediaInc
www.youtube.com/AmherstMedia
www.twitter.com/AmherstMedia
www.instagram.com/amherstmediaphotobooks

Contents

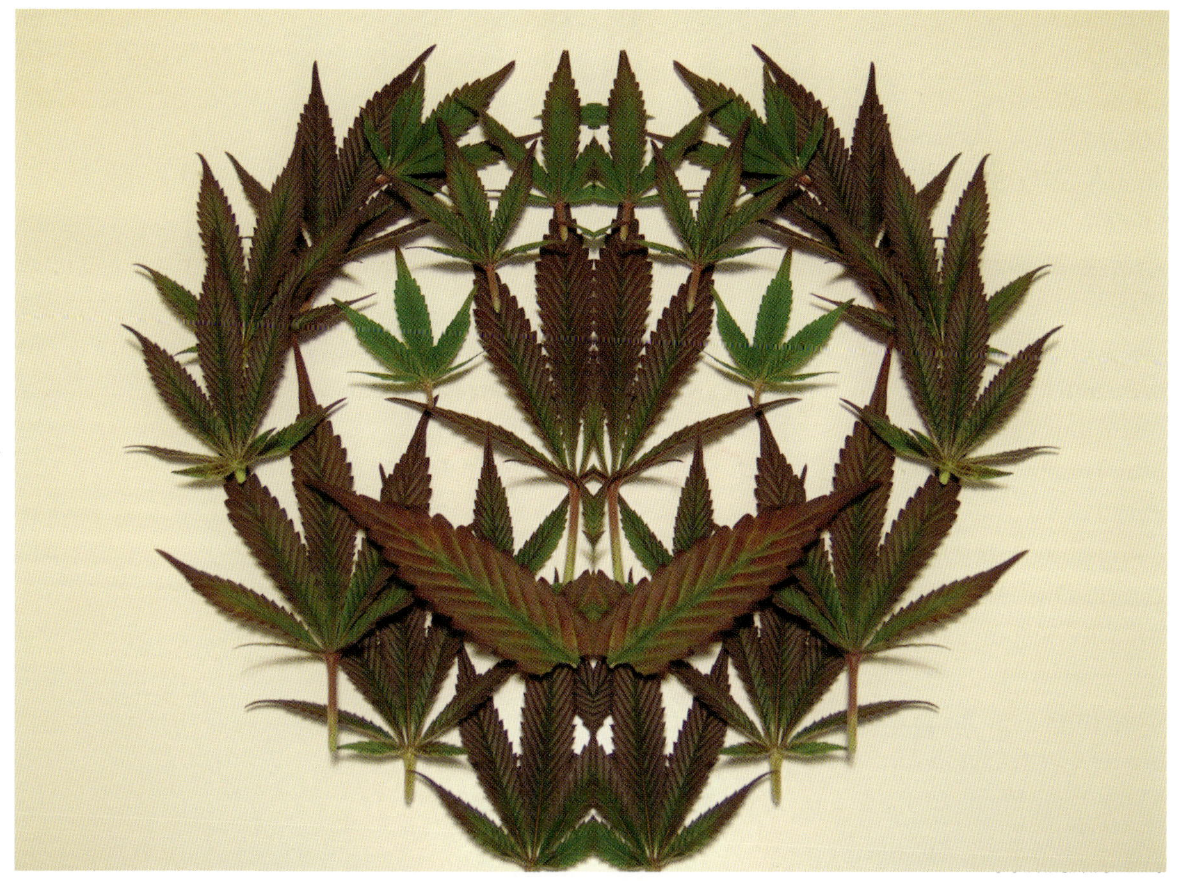

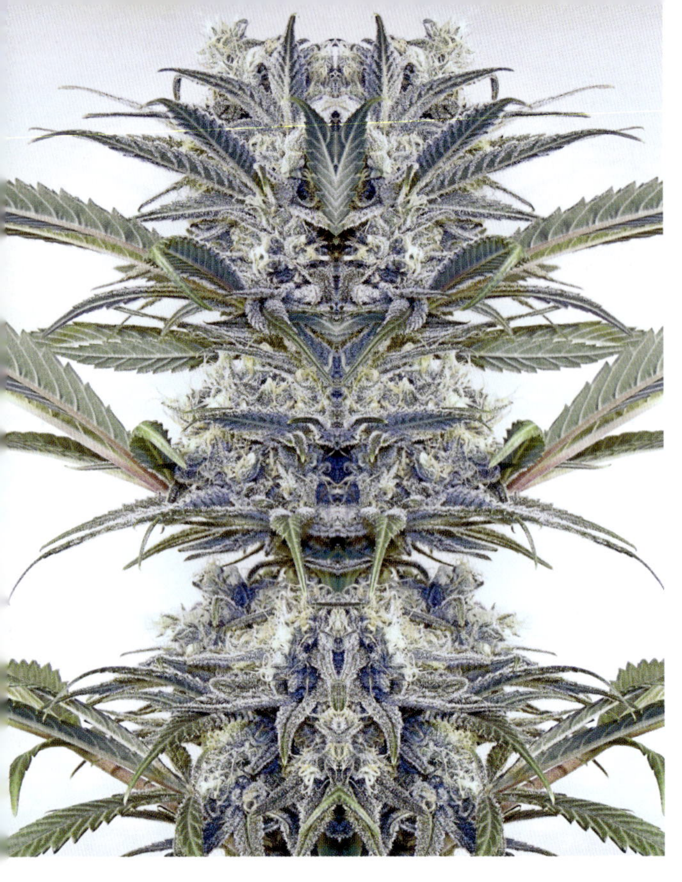

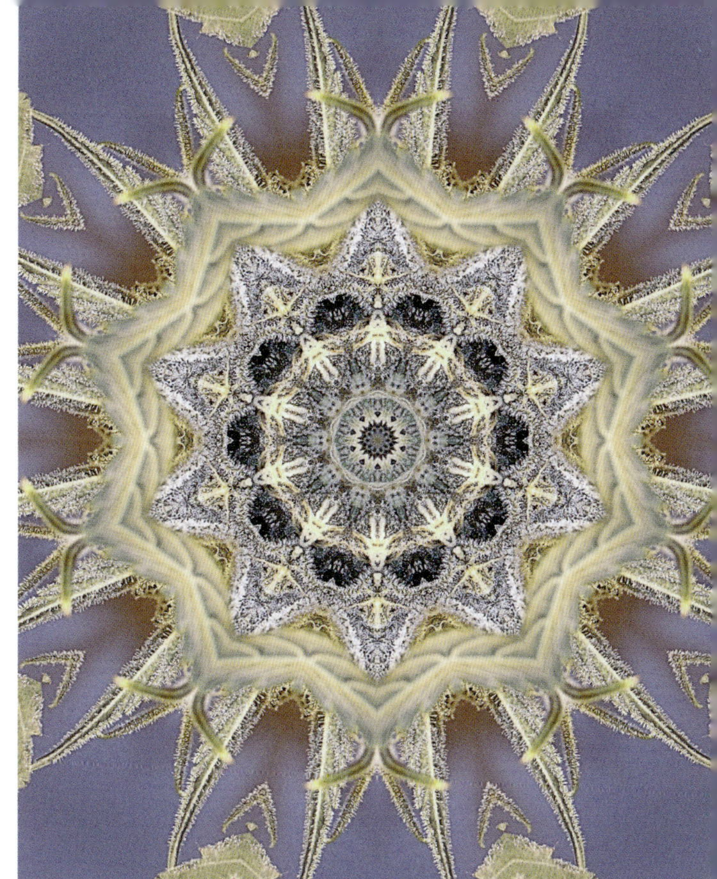

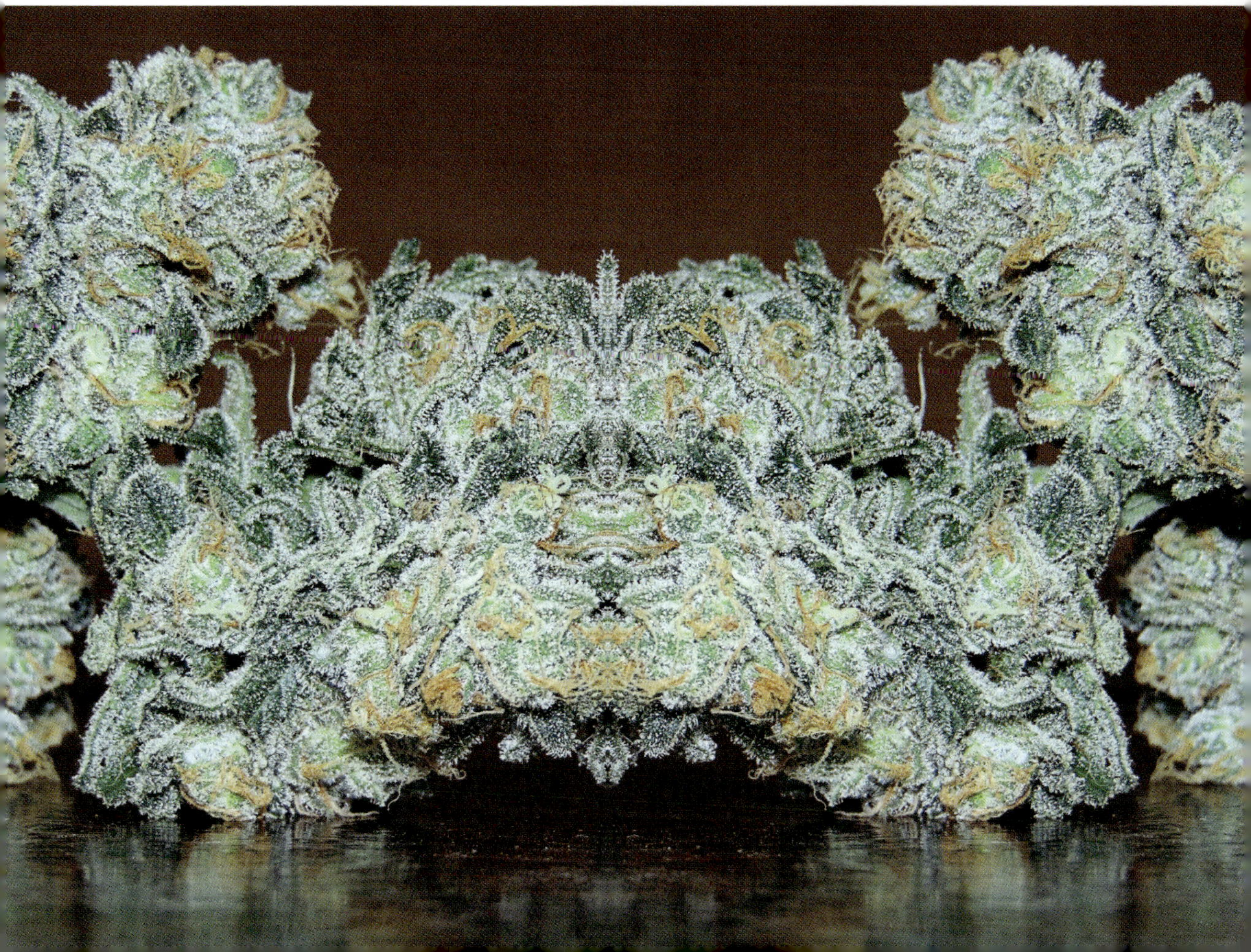

About the Author

Author Chris LaPrise grows his own cannabis for medicine and is an avid nature photographer who has been taking photographs for more than 40 years. He's happy to combine these skills in an art form he refers to as "cannatography." Chris cites that attending Hash Bash in Ann Arbor, Michigan, and uniting with like-minded people who rallied to challenge unjust marijuana laws have been memorable parts of his personal journey. He fondly recalls being able to smoke with Chef Ra (a long-time cannabis rights advocate and cannabis foods writer) and later met up with Ed Rosenthal (horticulturist, author, publisher, cannabis grower and advocate for the legalization of marijuana use) and Elvy Mussika (the first person ever to use federally grown marijuana to treat her glaucoma) while she was being pushed in her wheelchair by Ed. The website Civilized.life recognized Chris for "creating art that inspires," in Ophelia Chong's Unsung Cannabis Community Winners of 2017 list.

Acknowledgments

I would like to acknowledge the following people and groups that have inspired me over the years and encouraged me to "come out of the closet" in regards to cannabis.

I would like to thank Ed Rosenthal for his book, *The Closet Cultivator* (Quick American Archives; 2nd ed., 1999) and for his contributions to *High Times*. You taught me how to grow my own medicine during a difficult time in cannabis history—you *and* Mel Frank, I should say!

To my beautiful, loving wife of 28 years; thanks for being you and for letting me be me.

I'd also like to thank Ophelia Chong for being a mentor, a great promoter of diversity, equality, stigma deflation, and cannabis images. She is the shortest and best friend you can have in the cannabis space.

"I would like to thank the Cannabis Leaders in California for welcoming me into their group and allowing me to look in from the outside. What I learned from you was priceless.

To the active military and veterans of the United States: thank you for your service. A special thanks goes out to those veterans who are fighting for the right to attain legal access to cannabis as an alternative to the opioids they are often prescribed. I hope this fight is over soon.

To the people, families, and communities that were torn apart by the unjust laws enforced in the drug war. To those on both sides who died because of it. This was a war against minorities and filled—and continues to fill—the prisons with people and strip them of the right to vote.

To the medical cannabis community around the world. Despite current laws and pressure from the government, you researched anyway. I am proud of you! You're healing people and saving lives with cannabis.

To the parents of kids with cancer, autism, and other conditions: thanks for sharing your cannabis success stories with me and the media.

To NORMAL and all the other organizations that have been on the front lines for decades, speaking out against cannabis prohibition.

To all of you: I wish all the love, peace, health, and happiness you can possibly desire in our short time on earth.

Speaking of a short time on earth, I want to dedicate this book to my father. While I was wrapping up my first draft of the text, my father, the man who got me interested in photography, passed away. He had been excited to see the book, even though it's full of cannabis photos. He had accepted my use of and passion for the plant long ago. He'd met many people who used cannabis, and he said they were good people. I know he's proud of me and my choice to do something different from most photographers. He'd seen a few of my cannabis images and was able to enjoy some of my cre-

ative nature images, too. I sure wish he'd had the chance to see the final book. R.I.P., Dad.

—Chris LaPrise

Introduction

The collection of images in this book took a couple of years to create. Each one is unique. Making a great image is no easy task. In most cases, I captured four to twenty frames to get one that had something special, and good focus where it was needed. I used a tripod to help steady the camera for good, sharp, close-up detail and eliminate vibrations that could lead to image blur.

The lighting I used varied from image to image, too. Sometimes I used metal halide lights, other times it was fluorescent or high-pressure sodium lamps or the sun. Some of the photographs were made with mylar backgrounds. The curves and dents in it can reflect and bend light in different directions. Producing varying backgrounds is a must for this kind of photography, but at the same time, you need some continuity in case someone wants to display a cohesive grouping of images on their walls. This is one reason why I often create a series of images from one original image.

Mirrored images, kaleidoscopes, mandalas, faces, shapes, and beings await you as you turn the pages of this book. Most of the photographs should be viewed not only up close, but from a distance, too. A good piece of art will always attract you from a distance, and then draw you in for closer inspection. If I had a gallery, I would encourage people to stop and look at the images from six to eight feet away before approaching. This viewing distance allows one to see the image as a whole. I'd then encourage viewers to come closer, to view the fine detail, and the small faces, shapes, and beings within the artwork.

Set your imagination free as your browse through these pages. The greater your imagination is, or can become, the more you will love these images. Based on what I've witnessed, and others have noticed, too, everyone sees something different. Everyone has a unique interpretation. It's my hope that these images will be the impetus for many interesting conversations. Enjoy!

In the Begining

top—This image inspired me to look at cannabis in a way that is different than the way most people view it. I saw something that caught my eye and sparked my imagination. There was an eye in the center right, and part of a mouth below. I wondered, "What if I mirror this?"

bottom—So, mirror the image, I did. I was amazed at how close the face was to what I had envisioned. I was looking at the image as a whole, as most people do at first glance. Then I really looked into the image. Whoa! I saw more faces, shapes, and beings in there!

following page—It's time to set your imagination free.

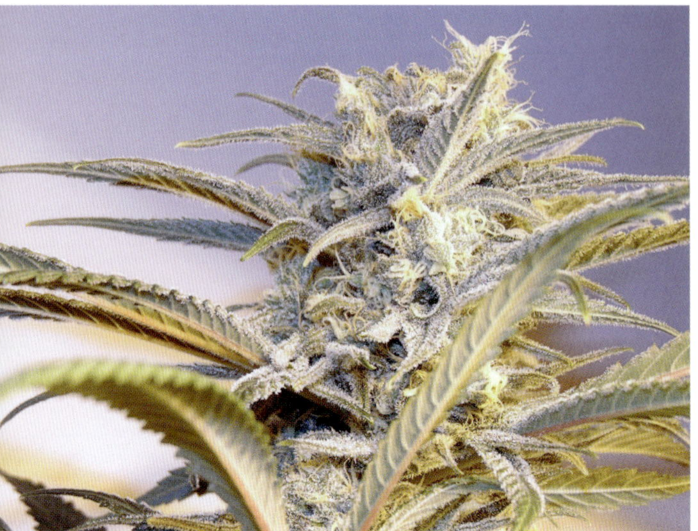

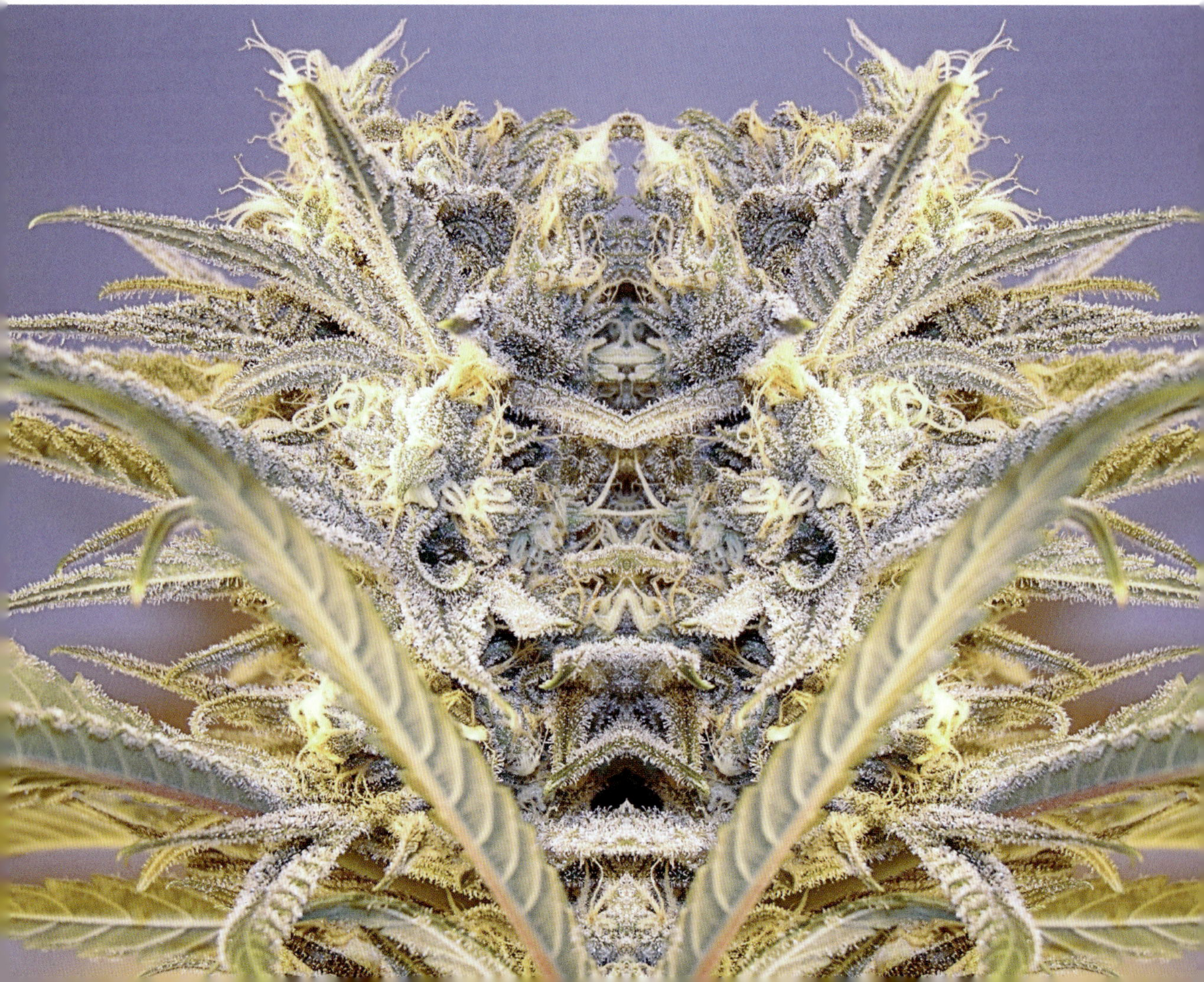

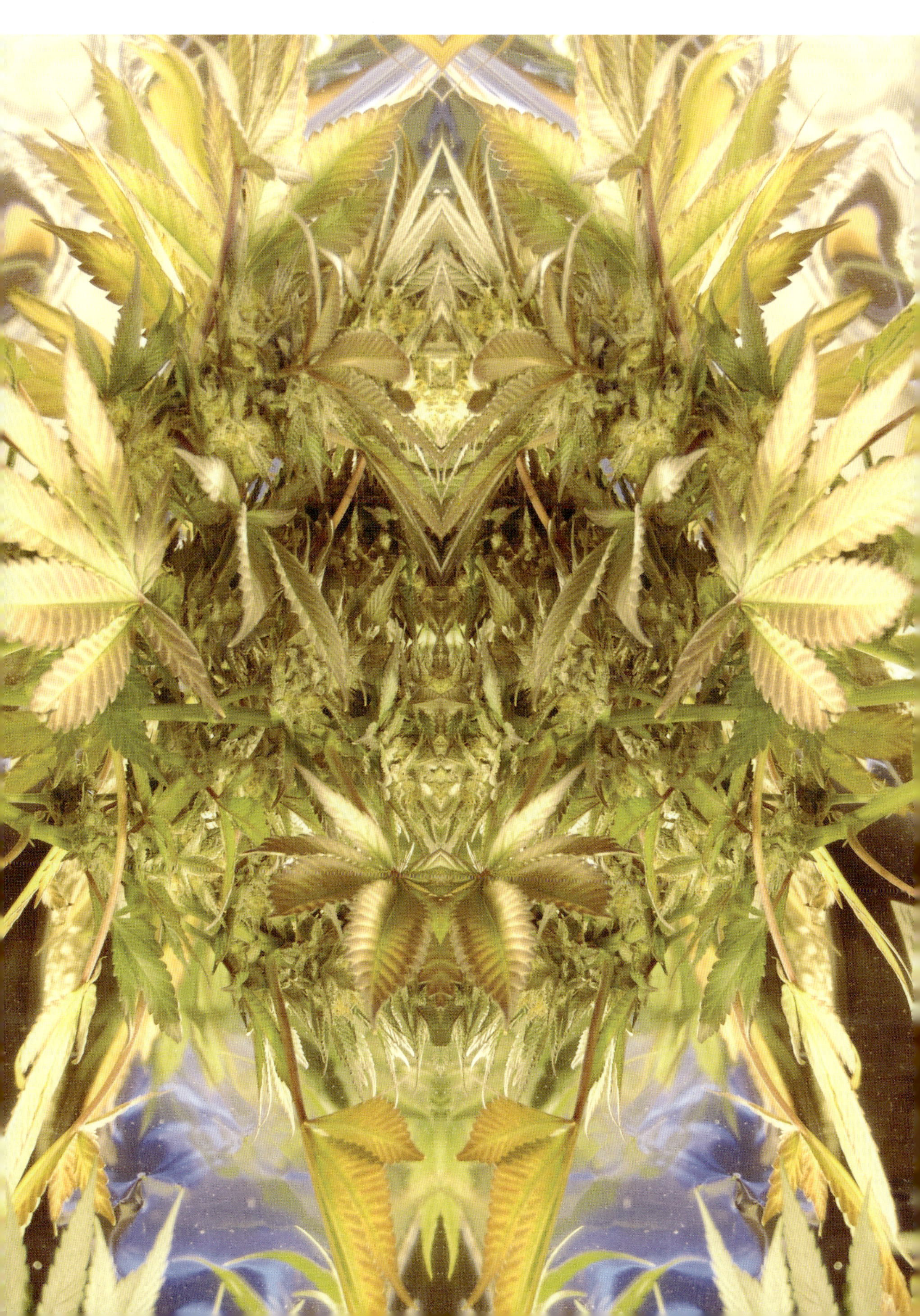

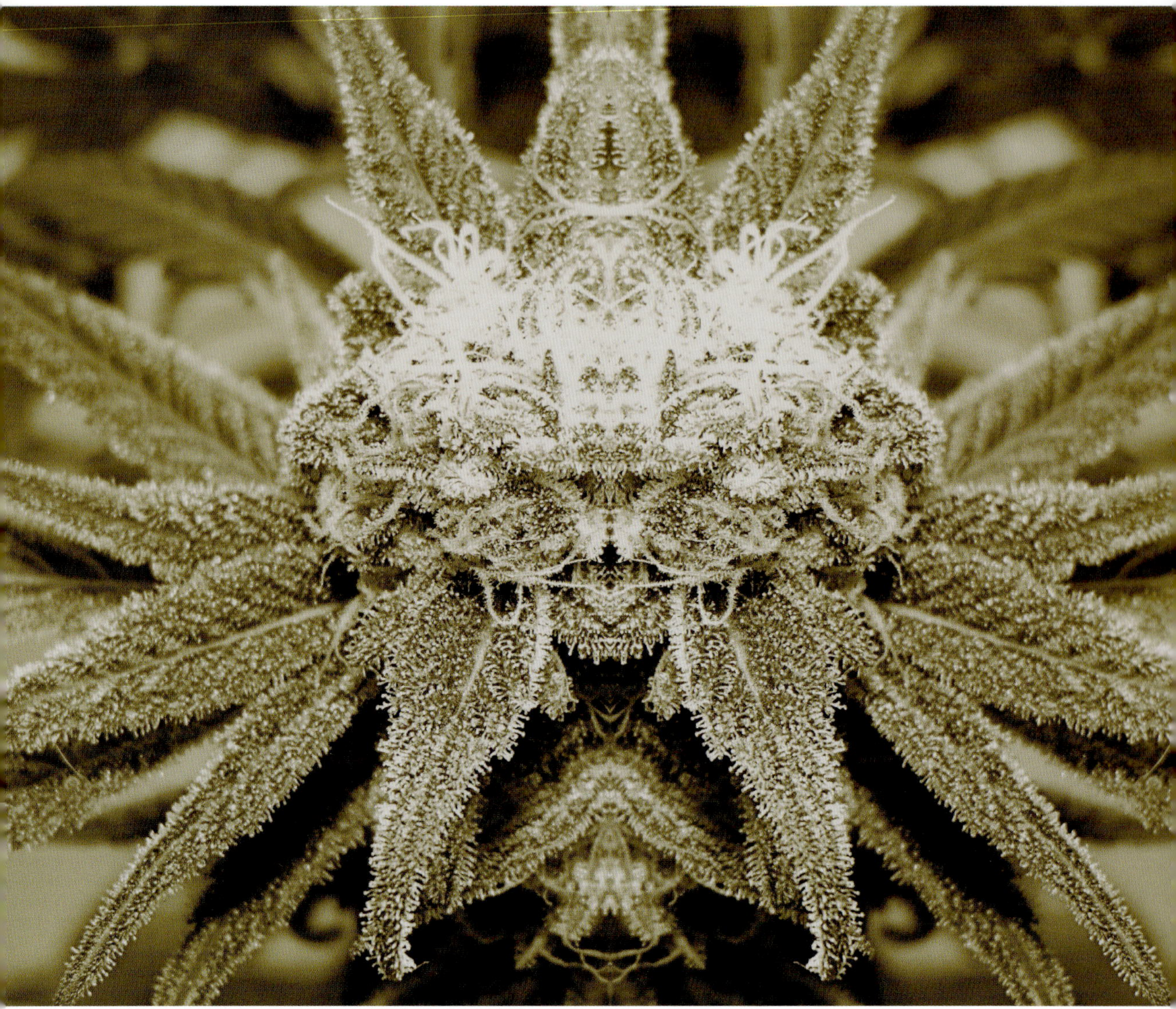

Canna-Cat

above—Mirroring became fascinating to me; so did macro photography. The buds, hairs, and trichomes are admirable and very photogenic, especially in macro. This image is called *Canna-Cat*.

Complementary

below—The black background looks good with the sepia tones in the globe. I love the way the leaves stretch as they wrap around the globe. I would love to have an acrylic paper weight like this!

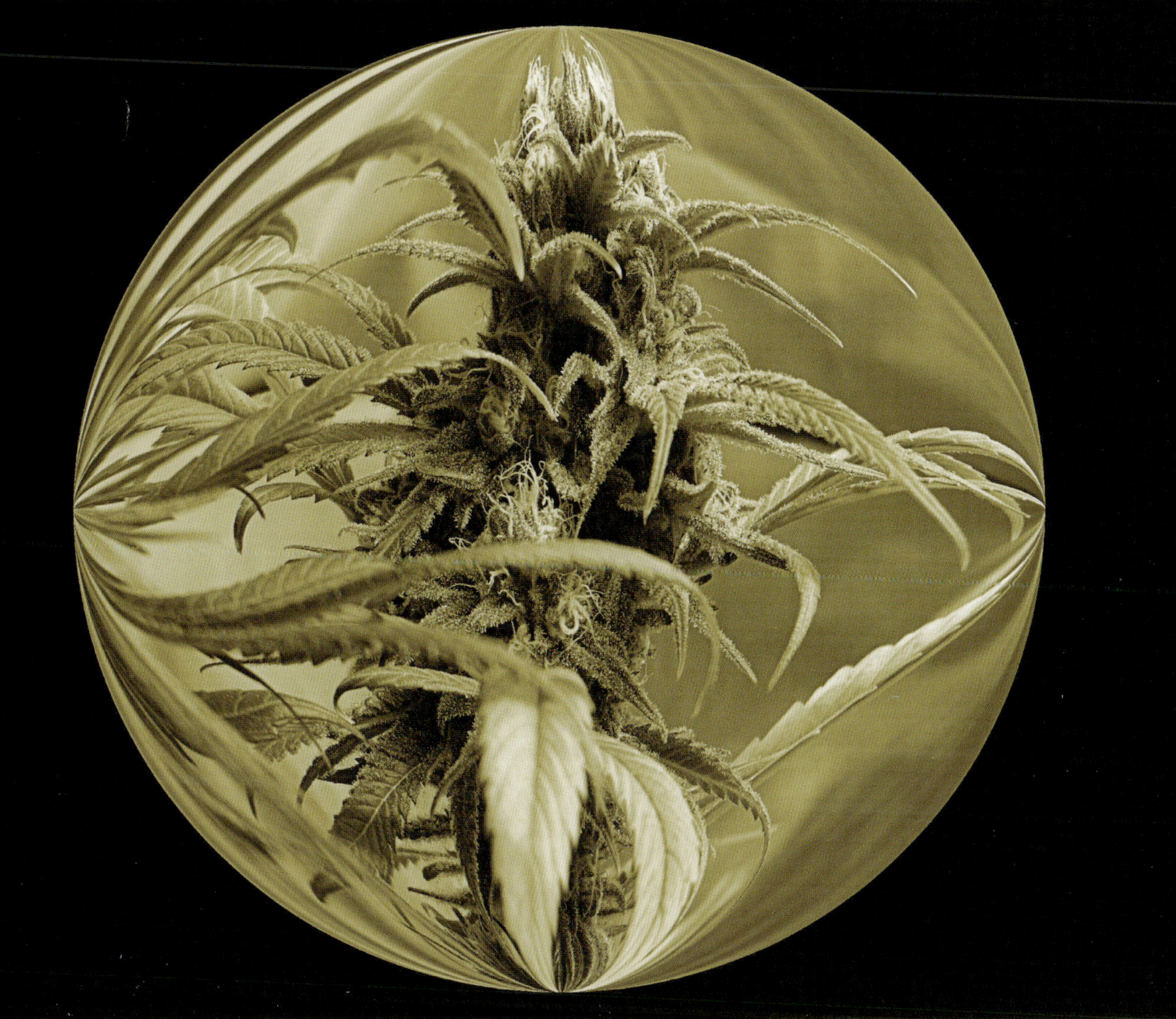

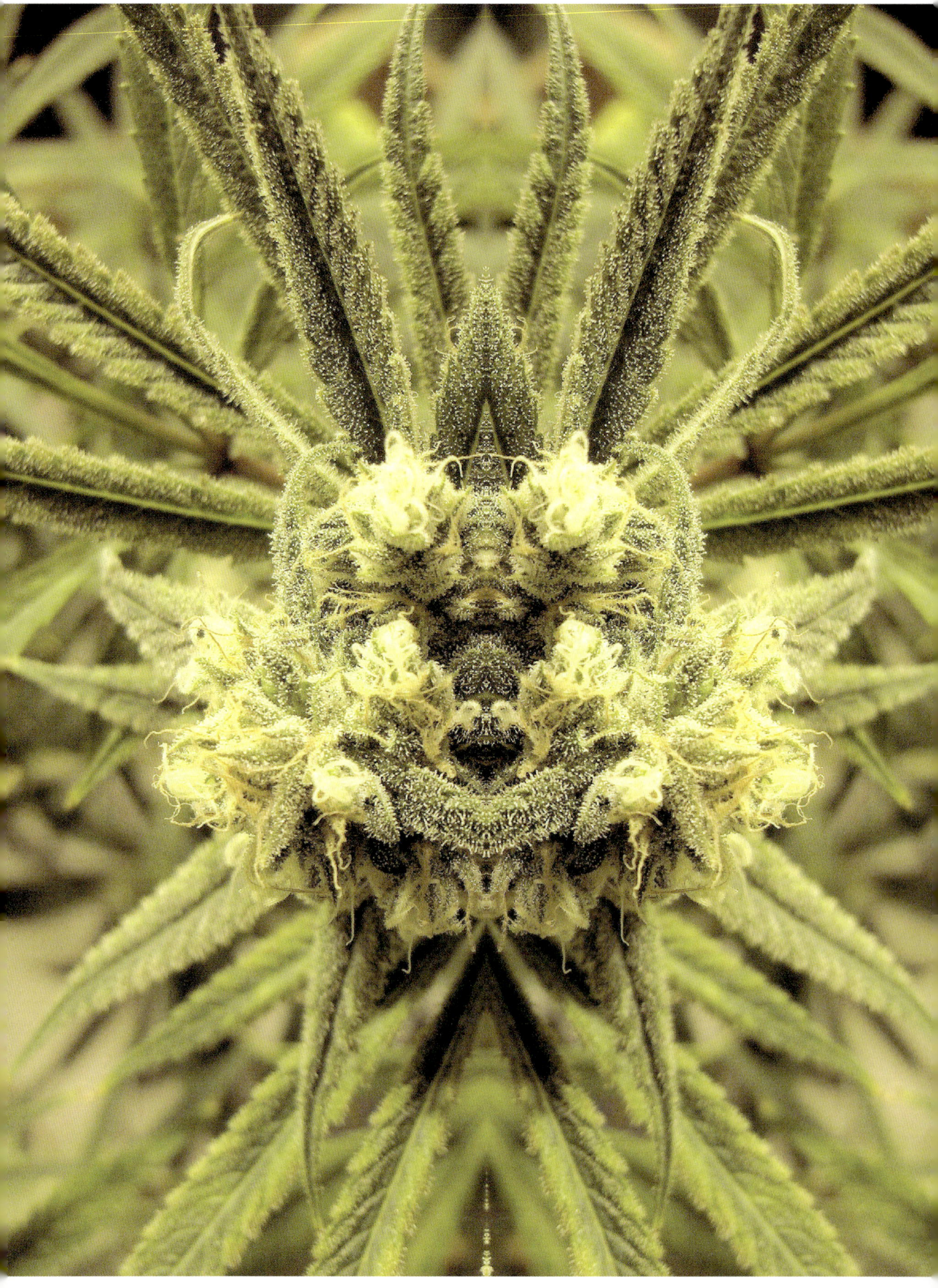

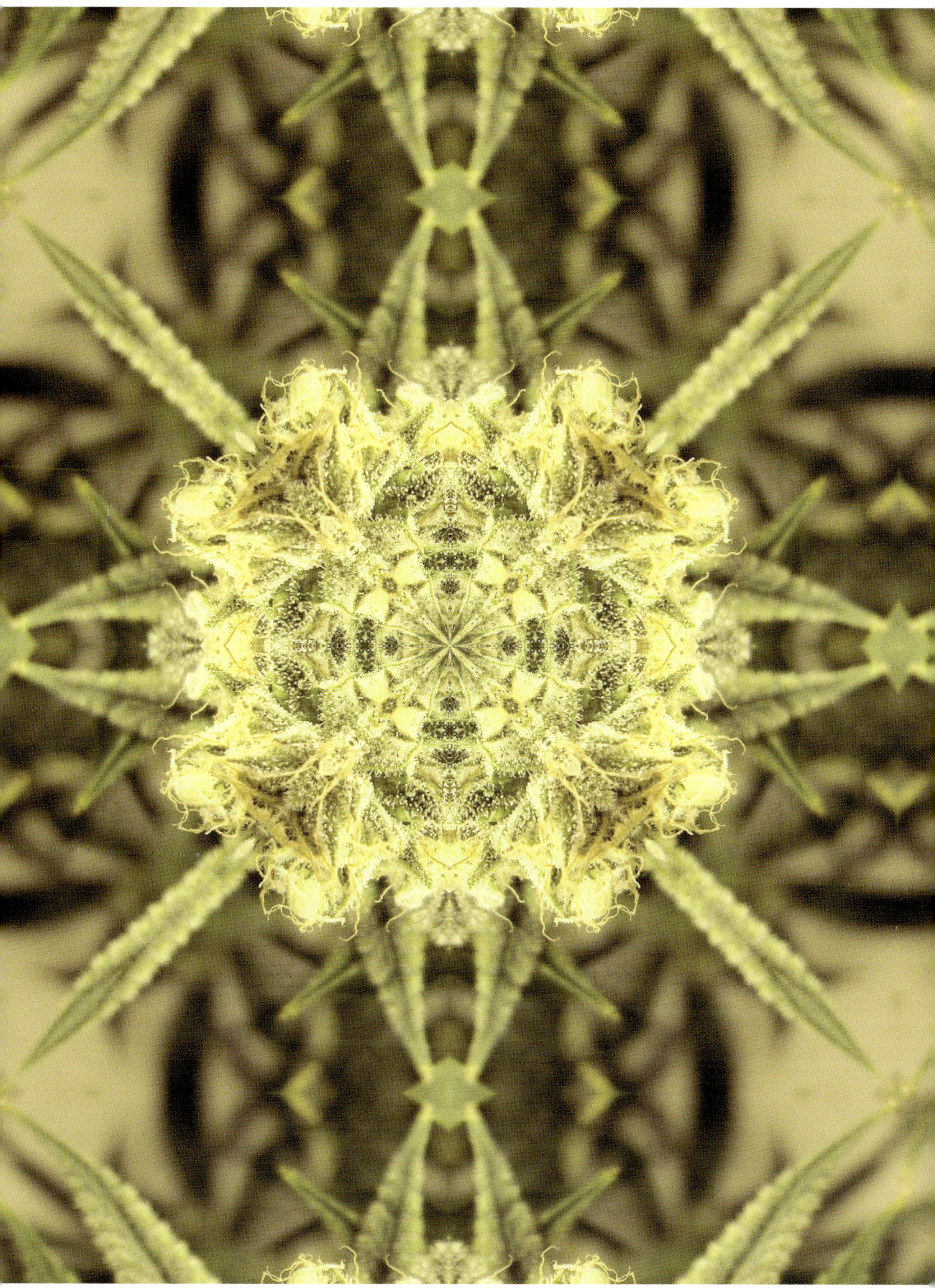

In Living Color

below—This image is one of my favorites. This is the original photograph, showing the actual colors of this plant. I did not alter the color at all. I added just a little light.

bottom—This is the same image, mirrored, in full size. I love the depth that mirroring the plant added. It created little caves that frame some really awesome creatures. As a whole, the plant resembles a muscular being with a large head, virtually no neck, and broad shoulders like a body builder. It reminds me of Ving Rhames flexing his muscles.

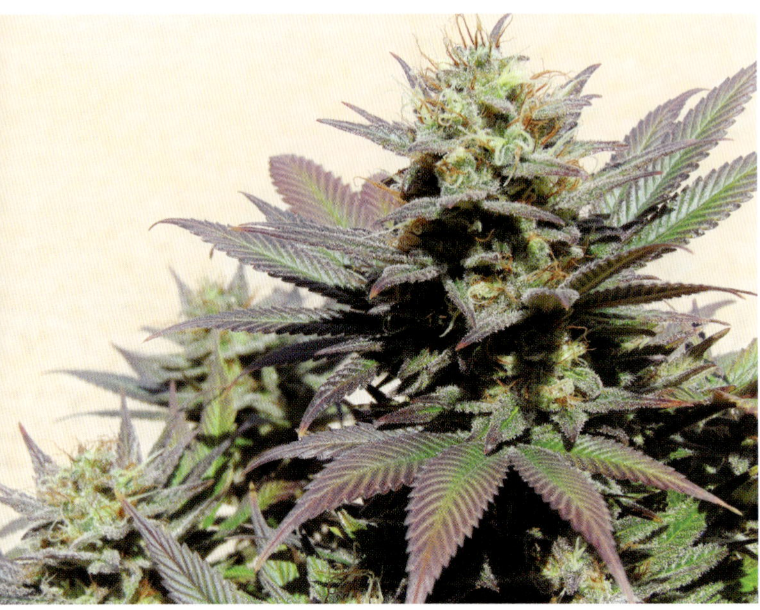

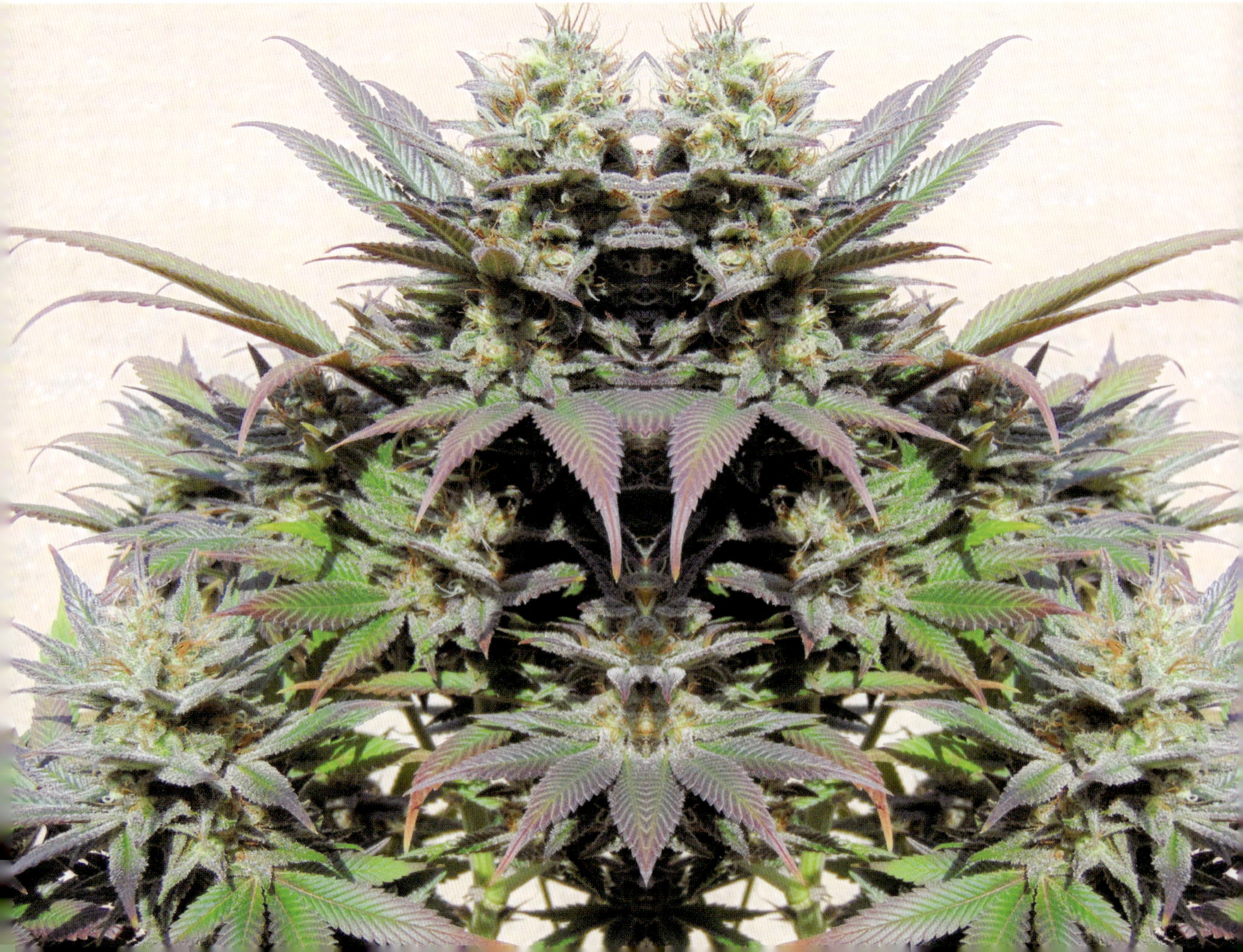

The Pistils

below—I zoomed in to one of the caves to capture the fine hairs coming off the pistils. You can see the difference between the receptive pistils and those that are waning and turning red, meaning they are no longer viable. It's a sign that the calyx is starting to mature. It also provides a better look at some nifty faces!

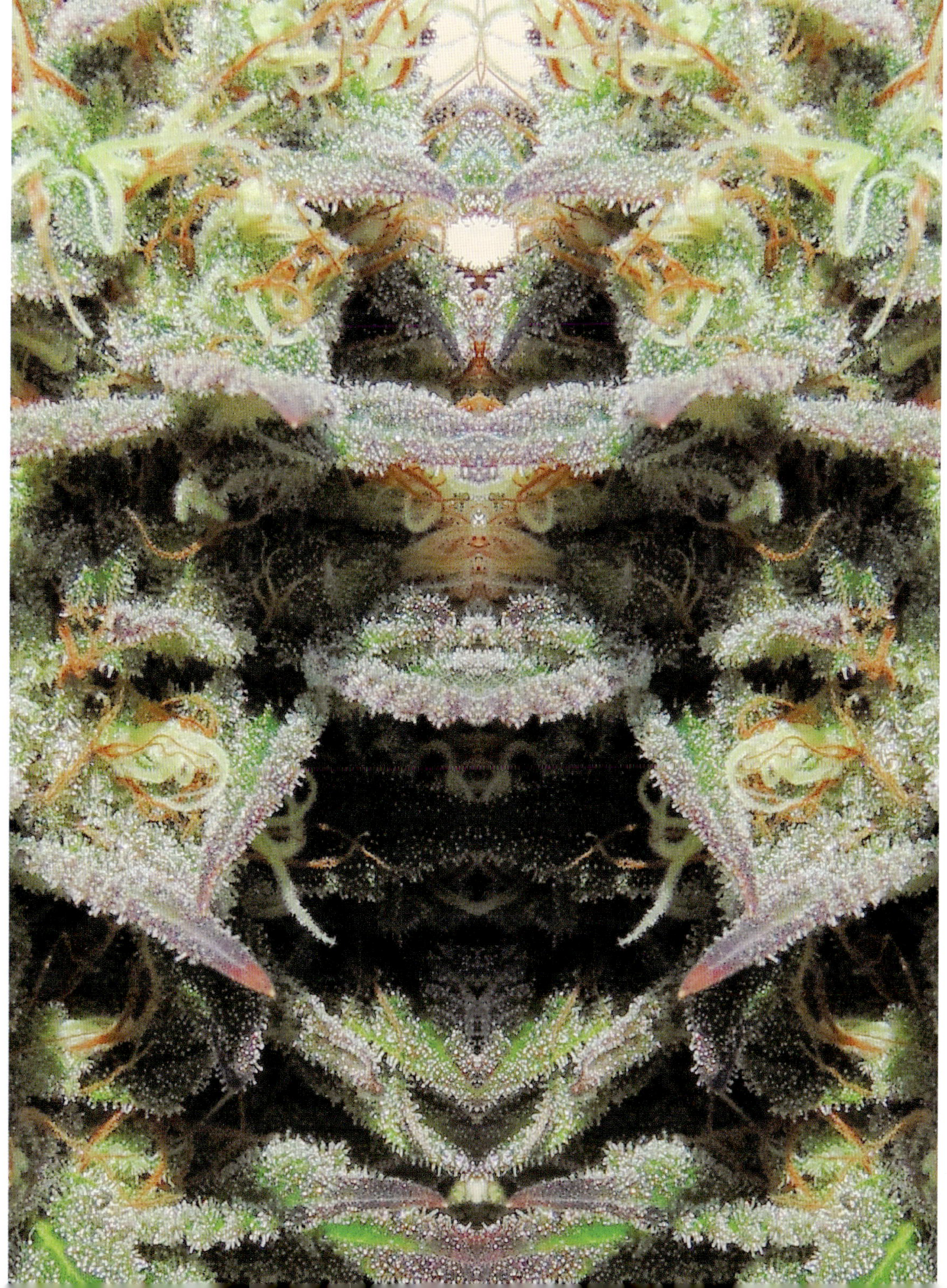

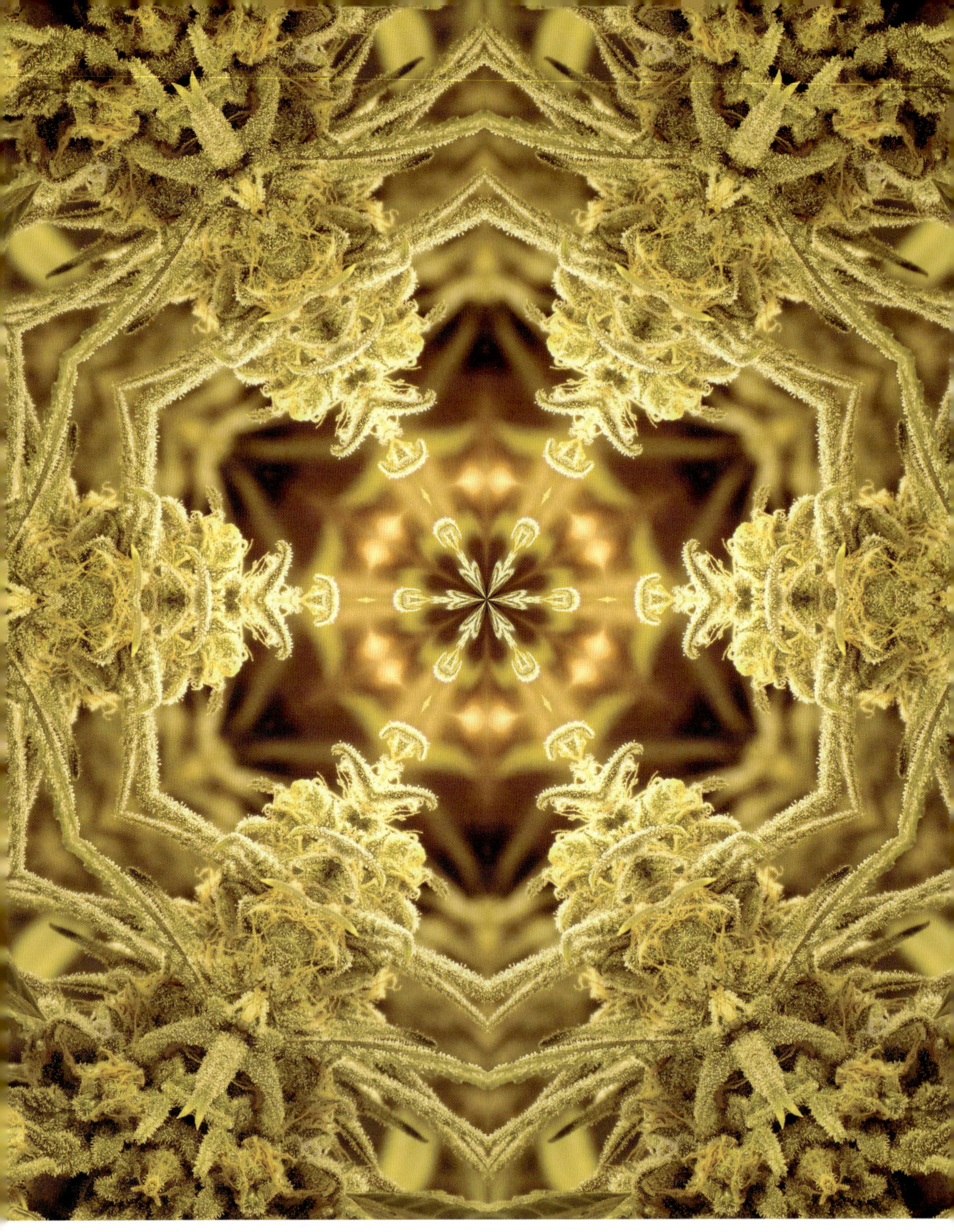

High Energy

above—These colas have combined and concentrated their power to produce energy pulses.

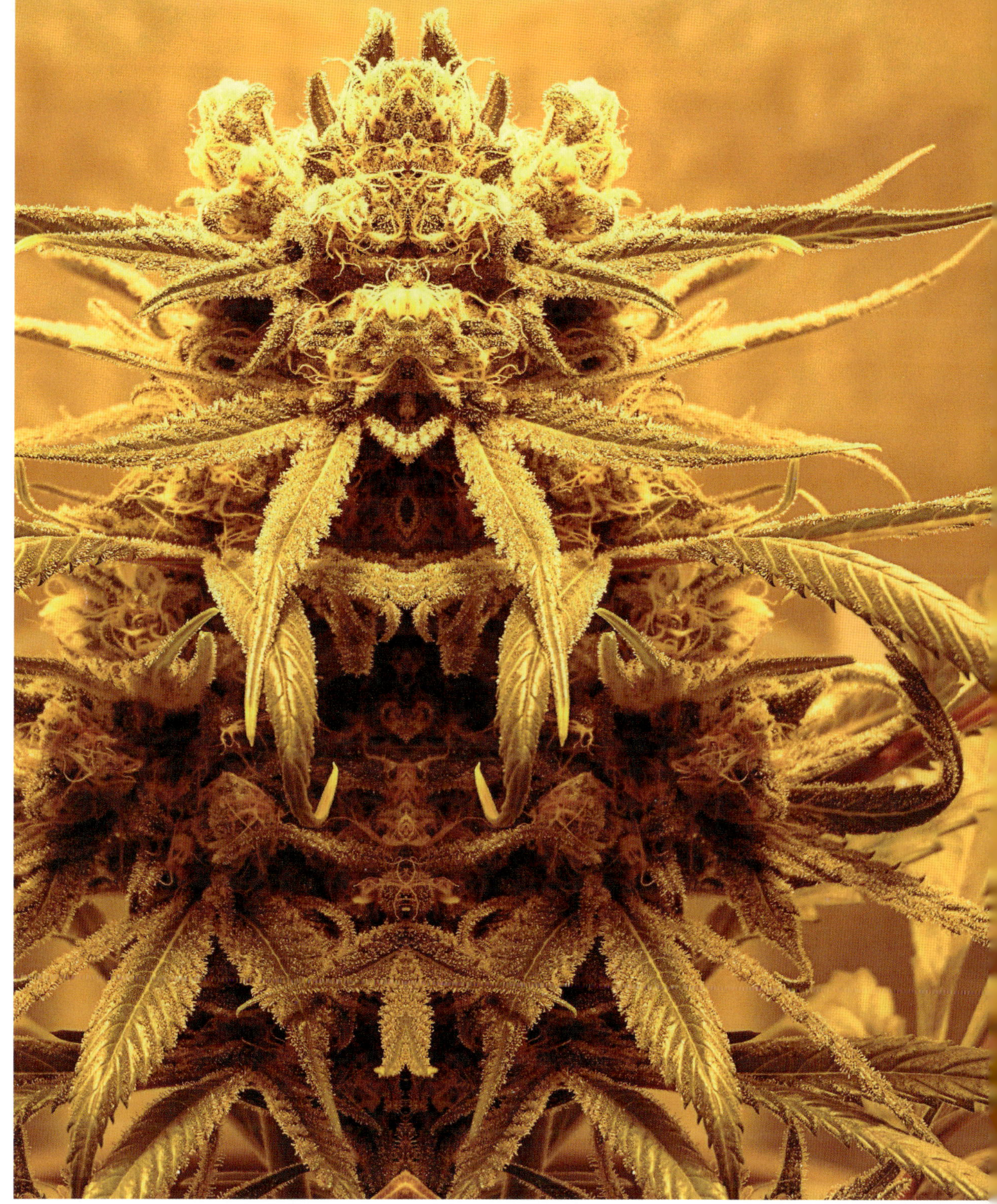

Cannasaurus Rex

above—The subject in this photograph has always reminded me of a dinosaur, so I named the image *Cannasaurus Rex*. I like to think that if it could make a noise, it would sound like Godzilla. This character has his high-pressure sodium camouflage colors on.

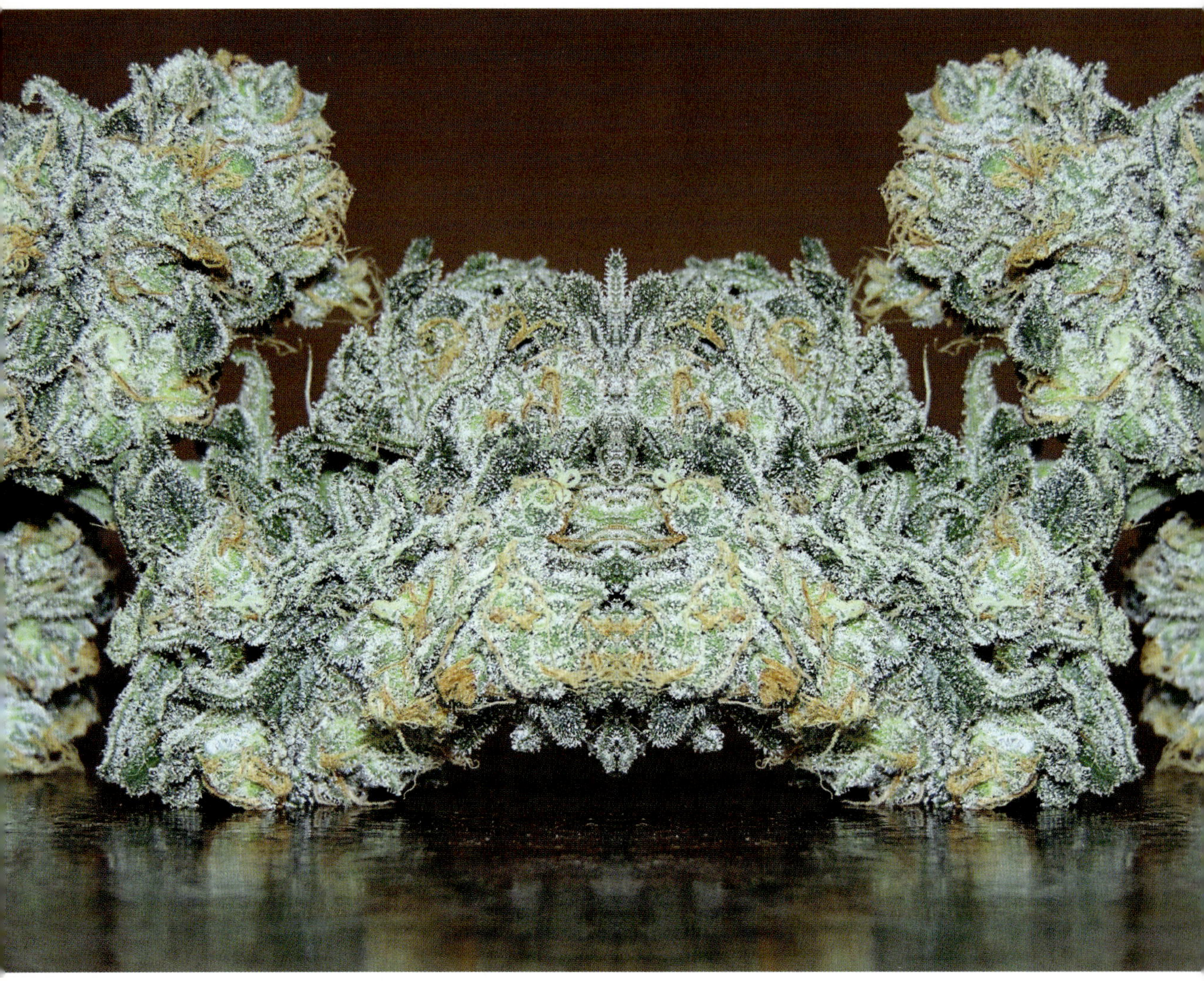

Blue Dream

above—This is the 2019 Blue Dream Super Coupe (modified class) in the pit stop at the Cannabis 500. Two bud mechanics marvel at the canna-car's body style and check for spider mites and mold before it hits the track again.

Canna-Birds

below—It's hard to not smile looking at this image. It's full of canna-birds with weed-leaf wings—and one has a big smile on its face. Various other trichome-covered canna-birds are following the happy one.

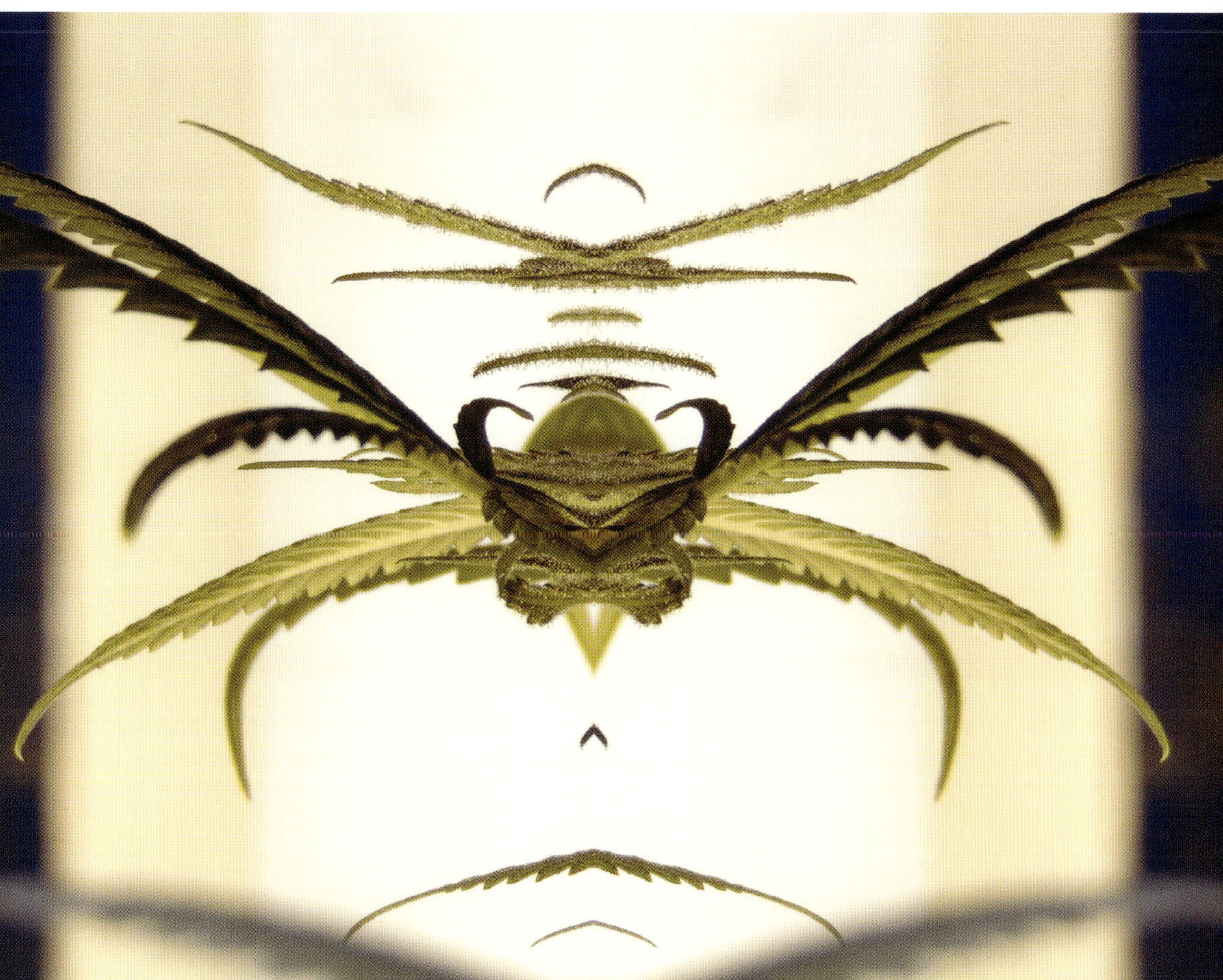

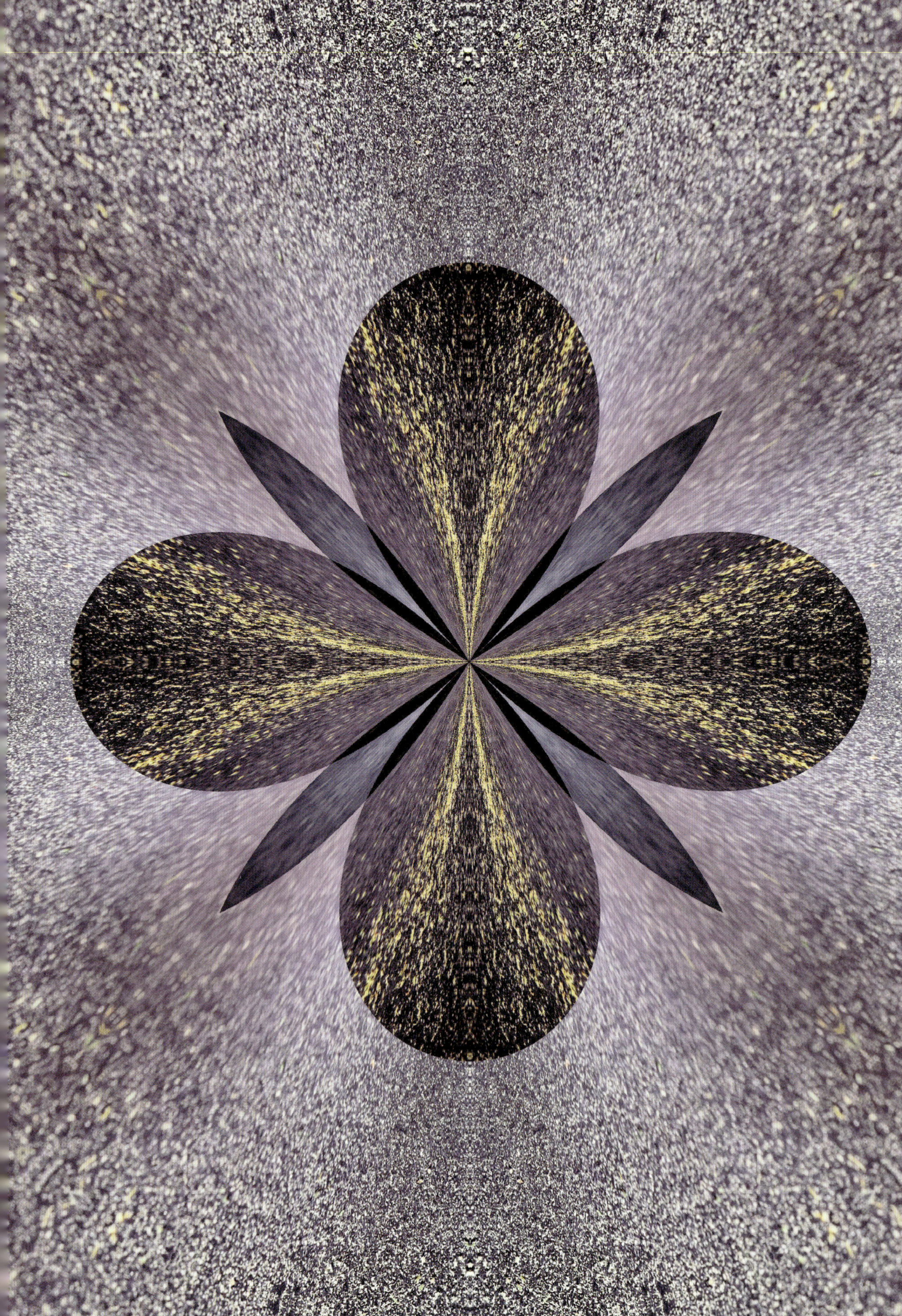

Just Kief

previous page—
This four-petal kaleidoscope is made of all kief on colored paper. I love how the two colors contrast. Kief comes from the bulbous heads of trichomes that contain THC, CBD, and other acids that are used for medical and recreational use.

right—This the kief I used to design the previous image.

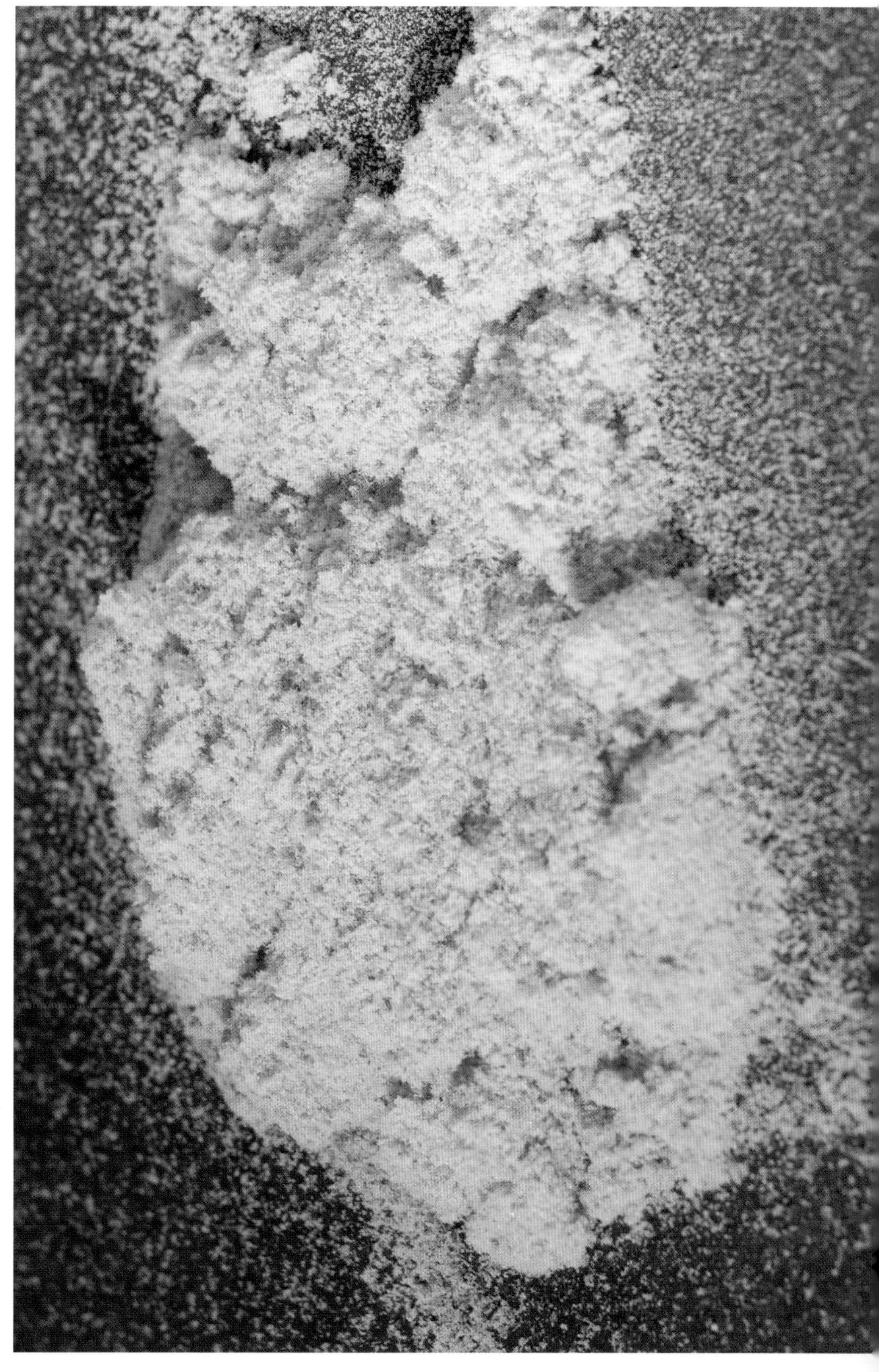

A Grand Old Flag

top left—I decided to play around with images I took in front of the flag. For some reason, I didn't like the look of the original shots. I don't know what bothered me about them, but there was something. I decided to take a different approach. I think this one would make a great image for canna-candy wrappers. Hint, hint.

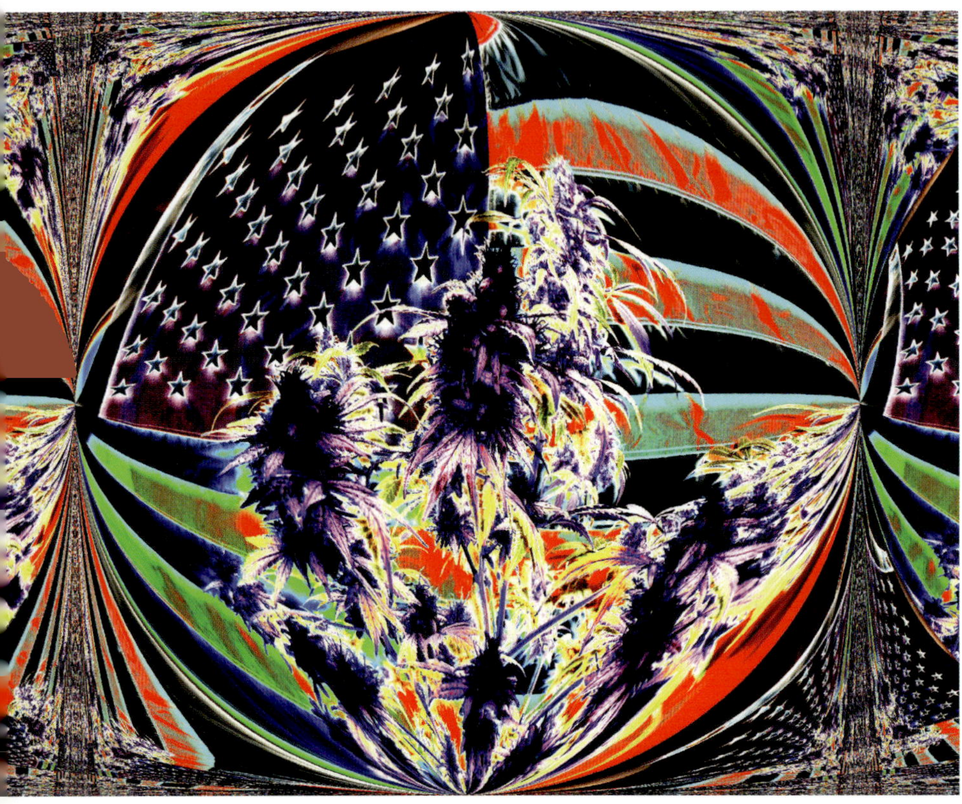

bottom left—On November 7, 2018, we woke up to great news. Michigan is the tenth state to legalize cannabis. We also have 33 states where medical marijuana is legal. Cannabis and the flag are uniting, and I am glad I lived to see the day.

following page—The leaves guide you to the center of this image, where you will find many faces, shapes, and beings. The guy in the orange frame with lines in it (just above the center) stands out to me. He reminds me of Smokey the Bear, complete with his hat and a smile.

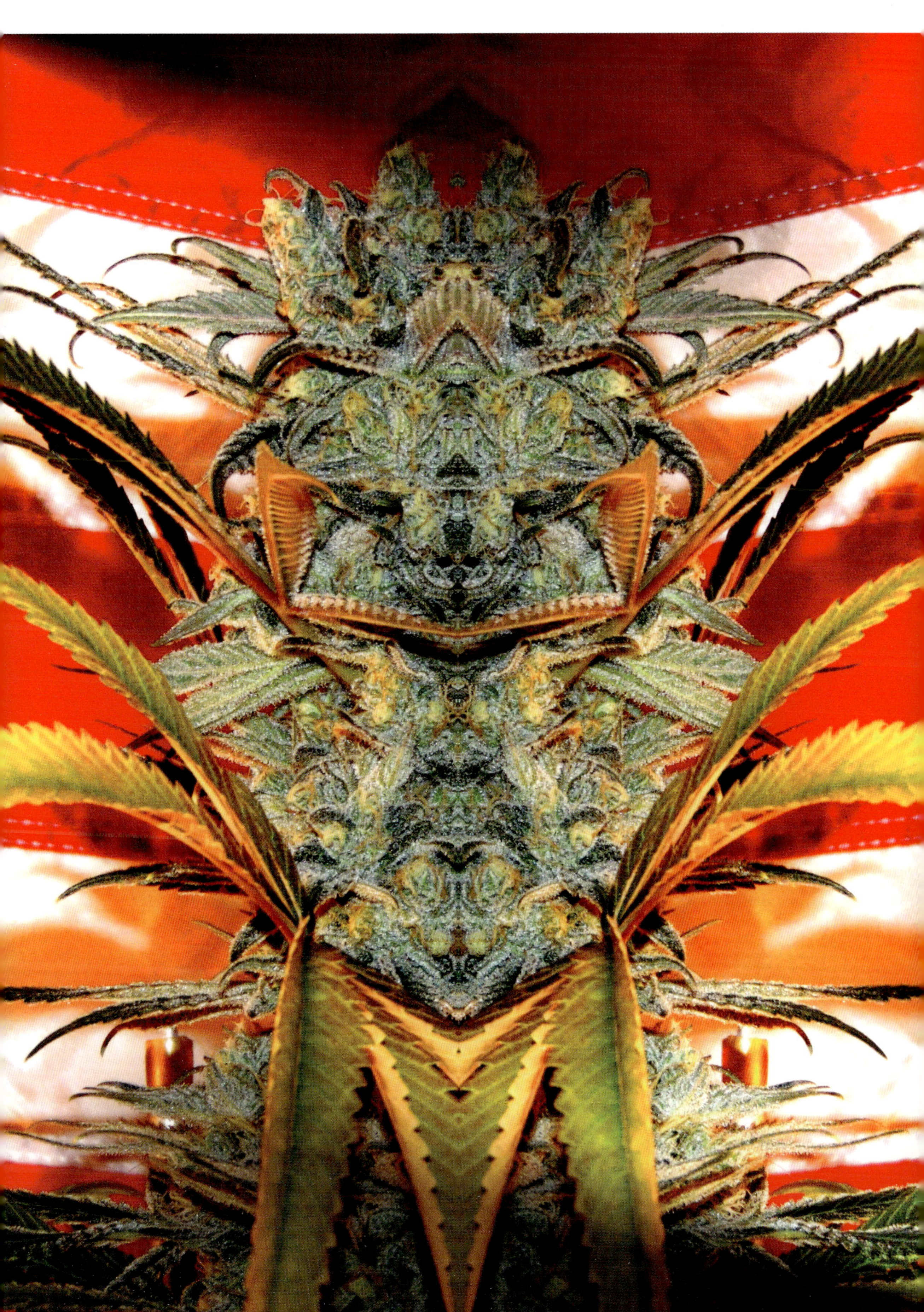

Stars, Sans Stripes

below—Here's another version of the globe with a reflection. We have an immature bud with stars, but no stripes. HPS (high-pressure sodium) lighting was used.

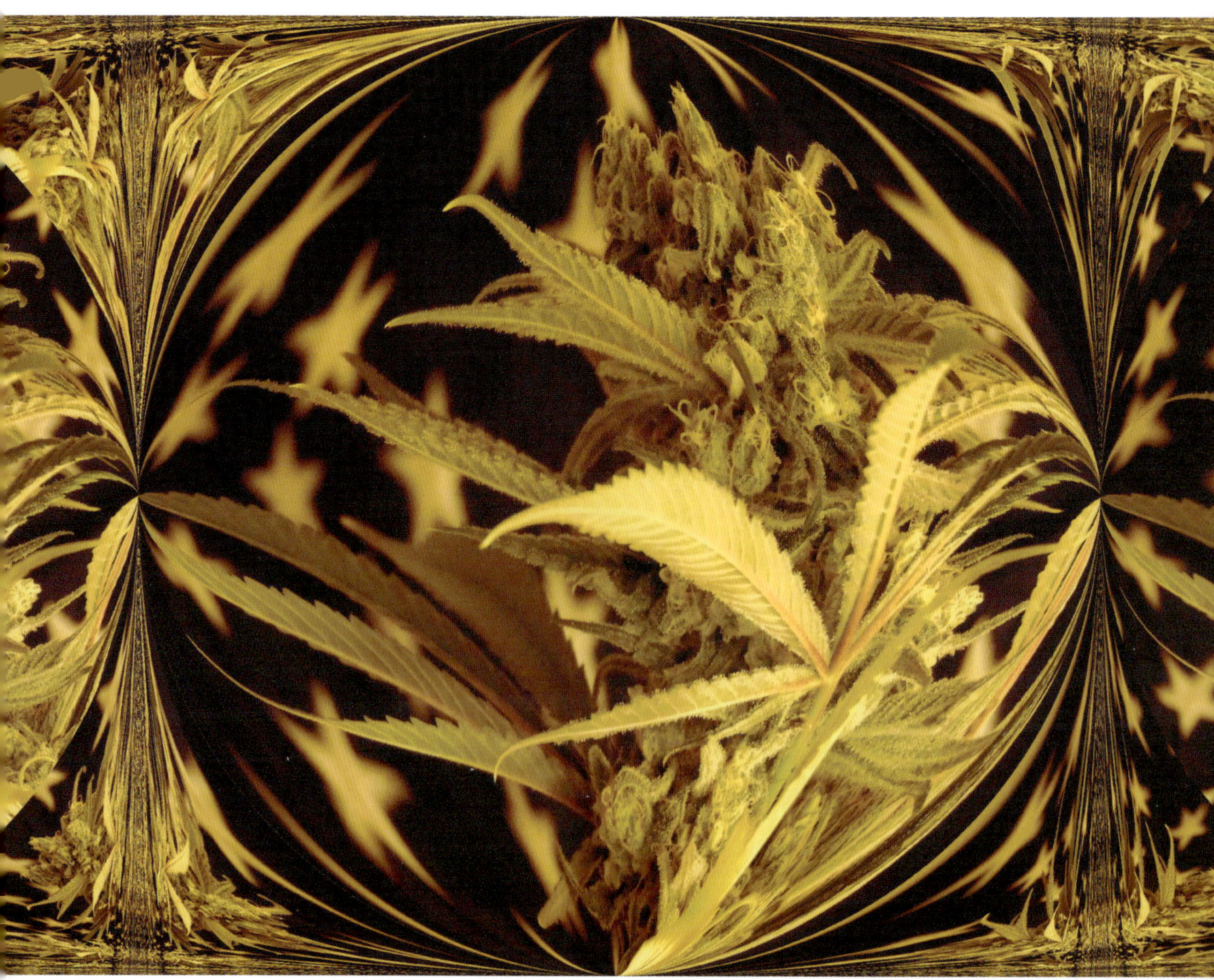

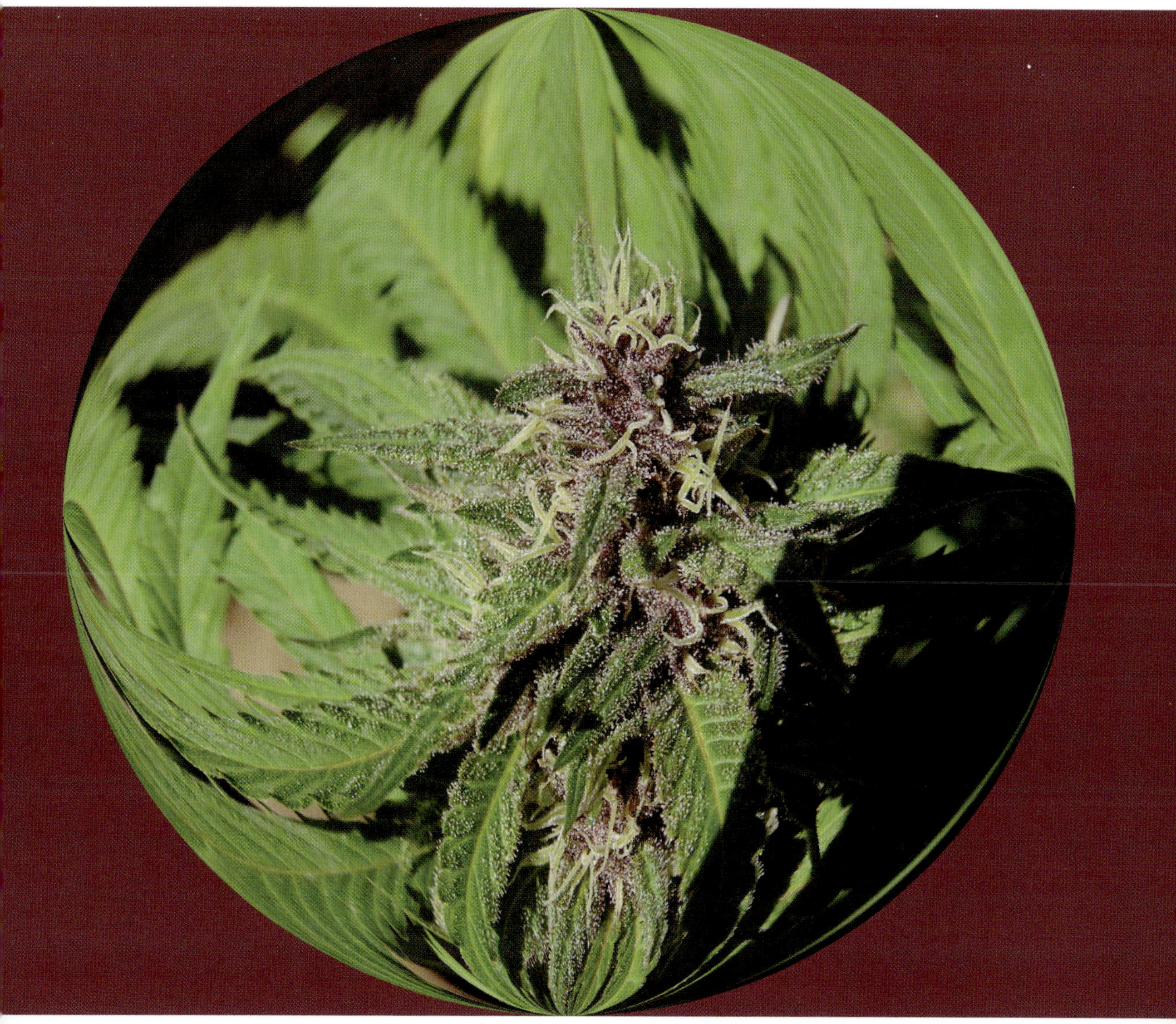

Adding Color

above—This is Blue Dream (full sun), in a globe with no reflection. I can make the background any color that is contained in the image by sampling the desired hue with the eyedropper tool in postproduction. It selects a single pixel from the image to create the color from. I use the Fill tool to paint around the globe, filling the background with color.

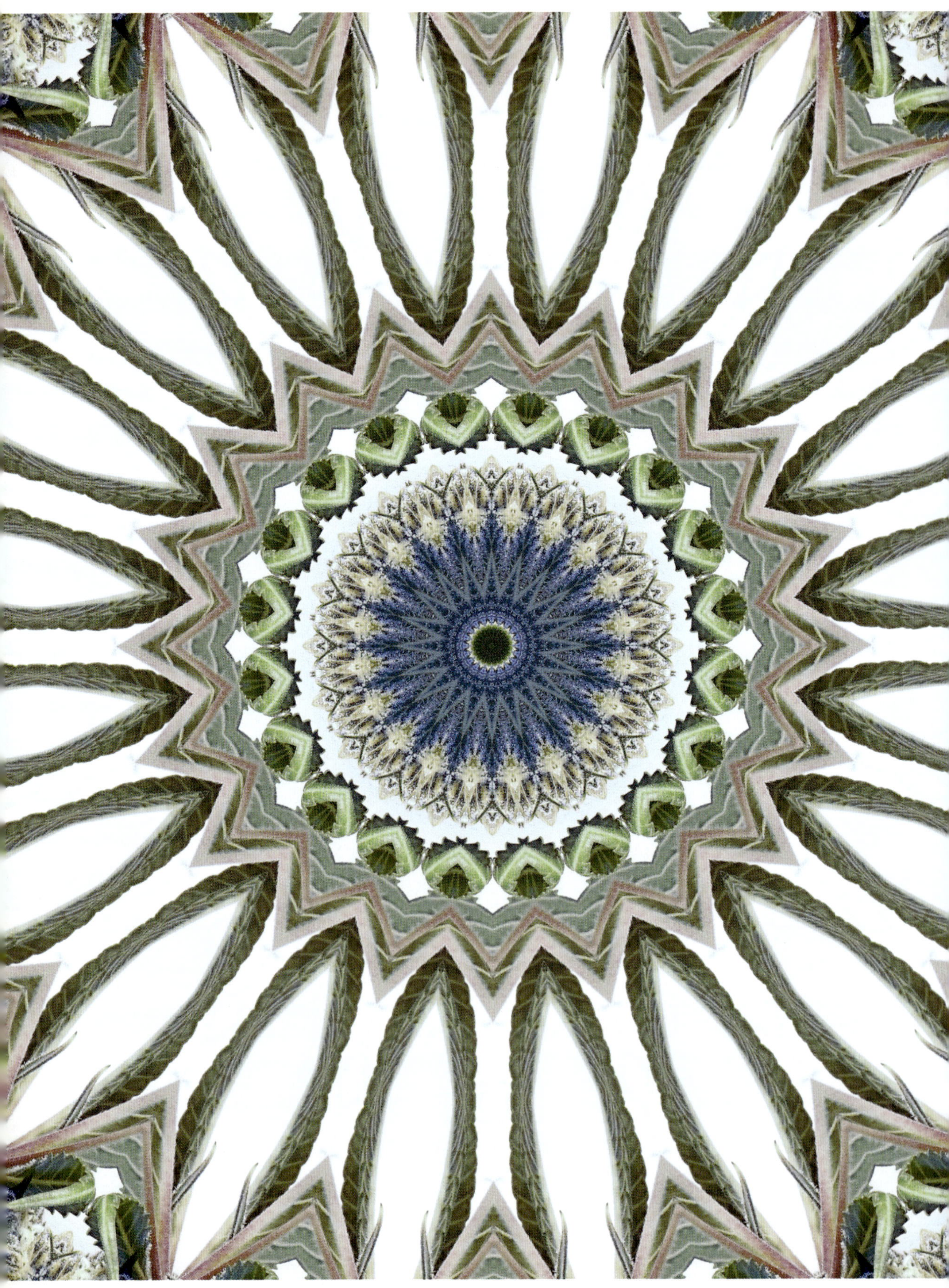

Ethnic
Flair

previous page—Twenty-petal leaf mandala.

top—Using mylar for the background added a nice, soft effect here. The eyes that appear in the bottom third of the image really jump out to me. They guide you to the nose and open mouth below. Combine that with the leaves spreading to the bottom of the frame, representing arms, and the claw-like hands above, and it looks like a strange being about to remove its giant, budded headdress.

bottom—This is the same image shown above, but made into a five-petal kaleidoscope. The stars that appeared took me by surprise.

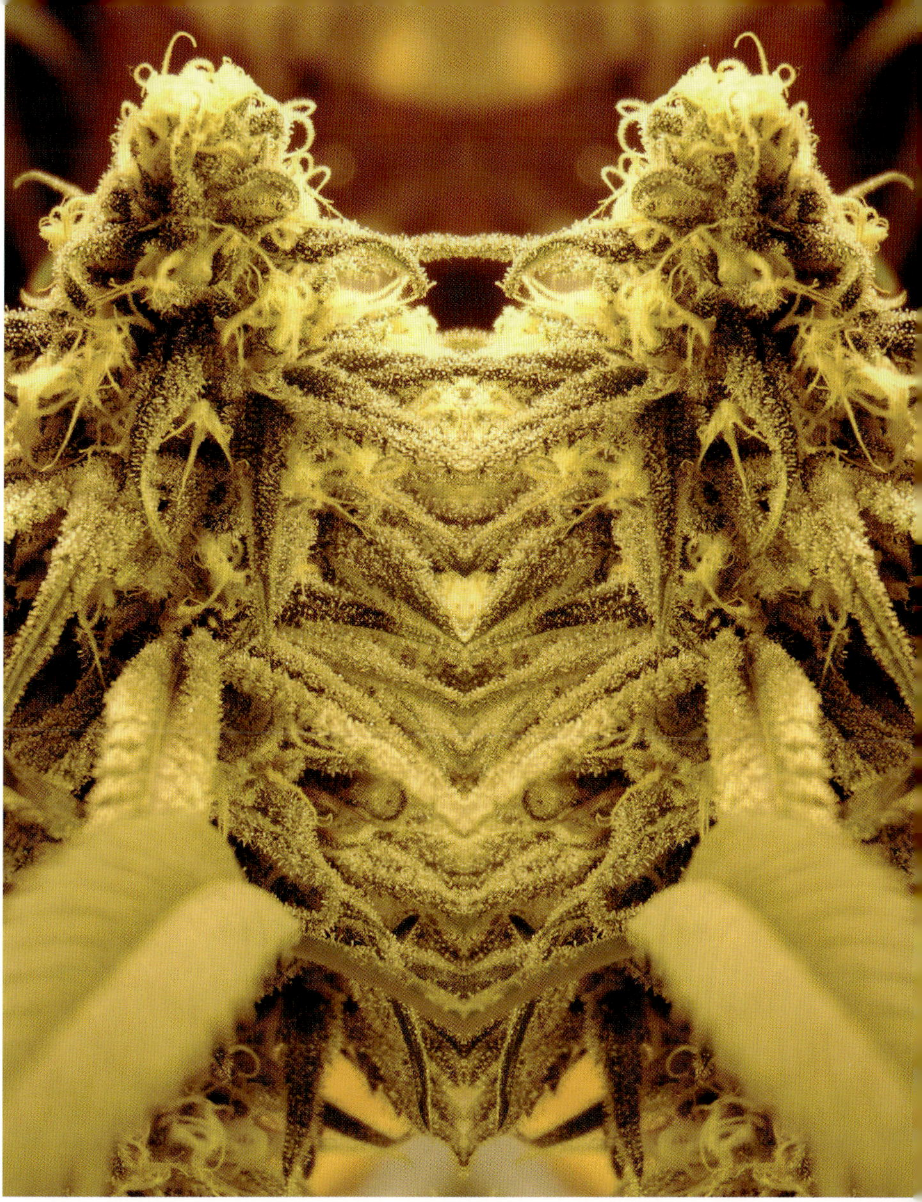

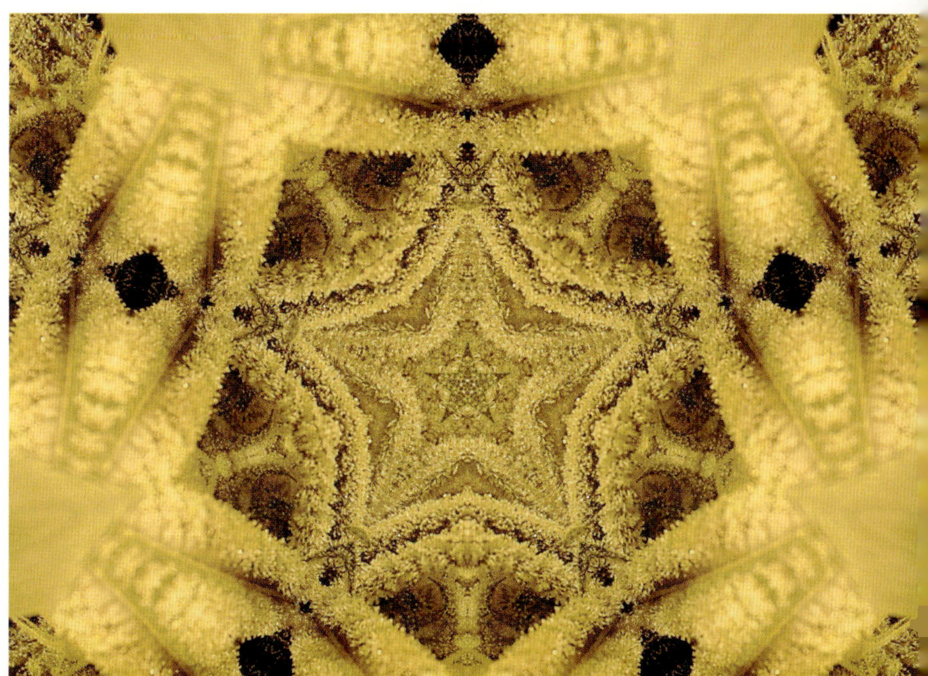

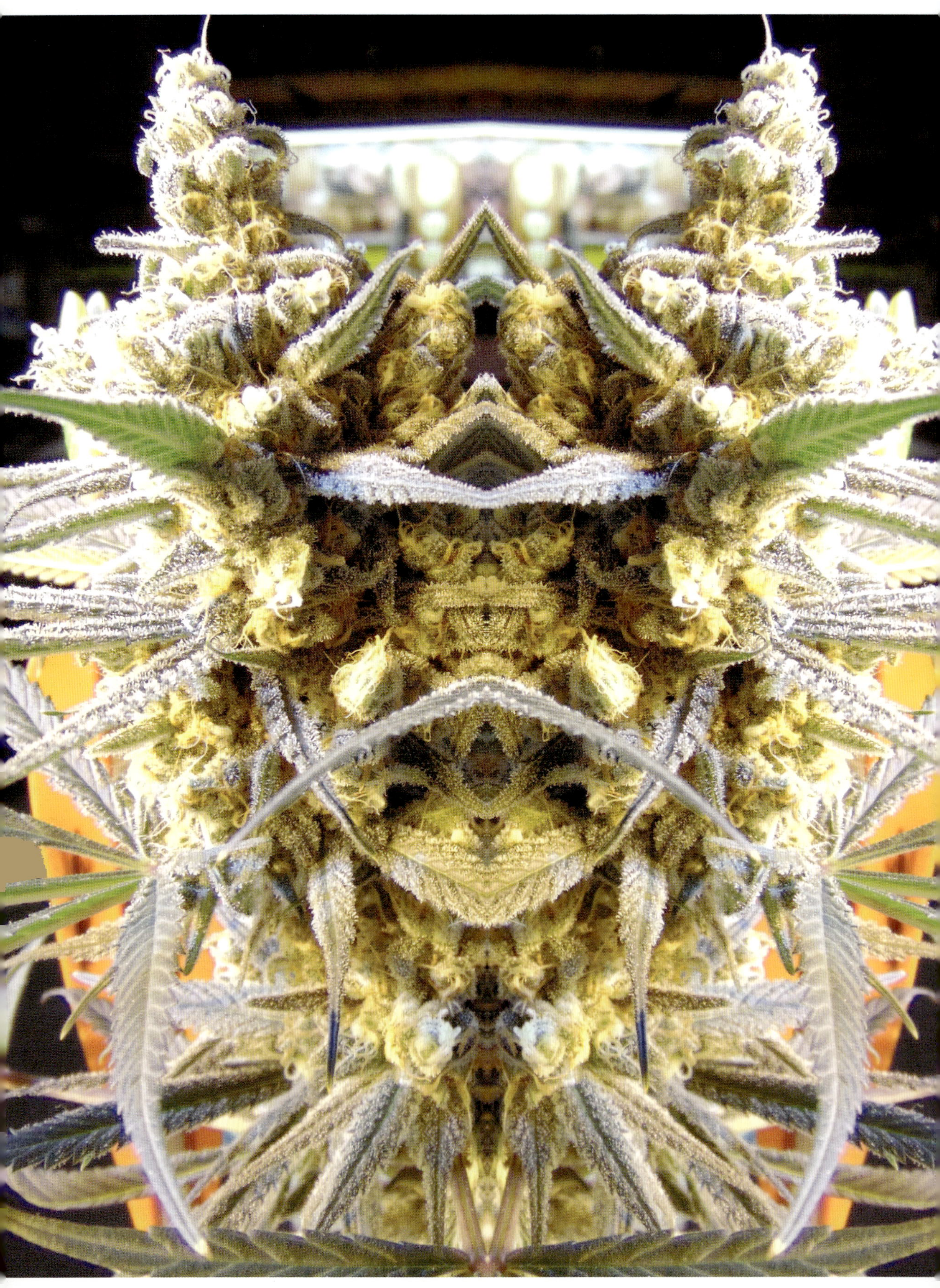

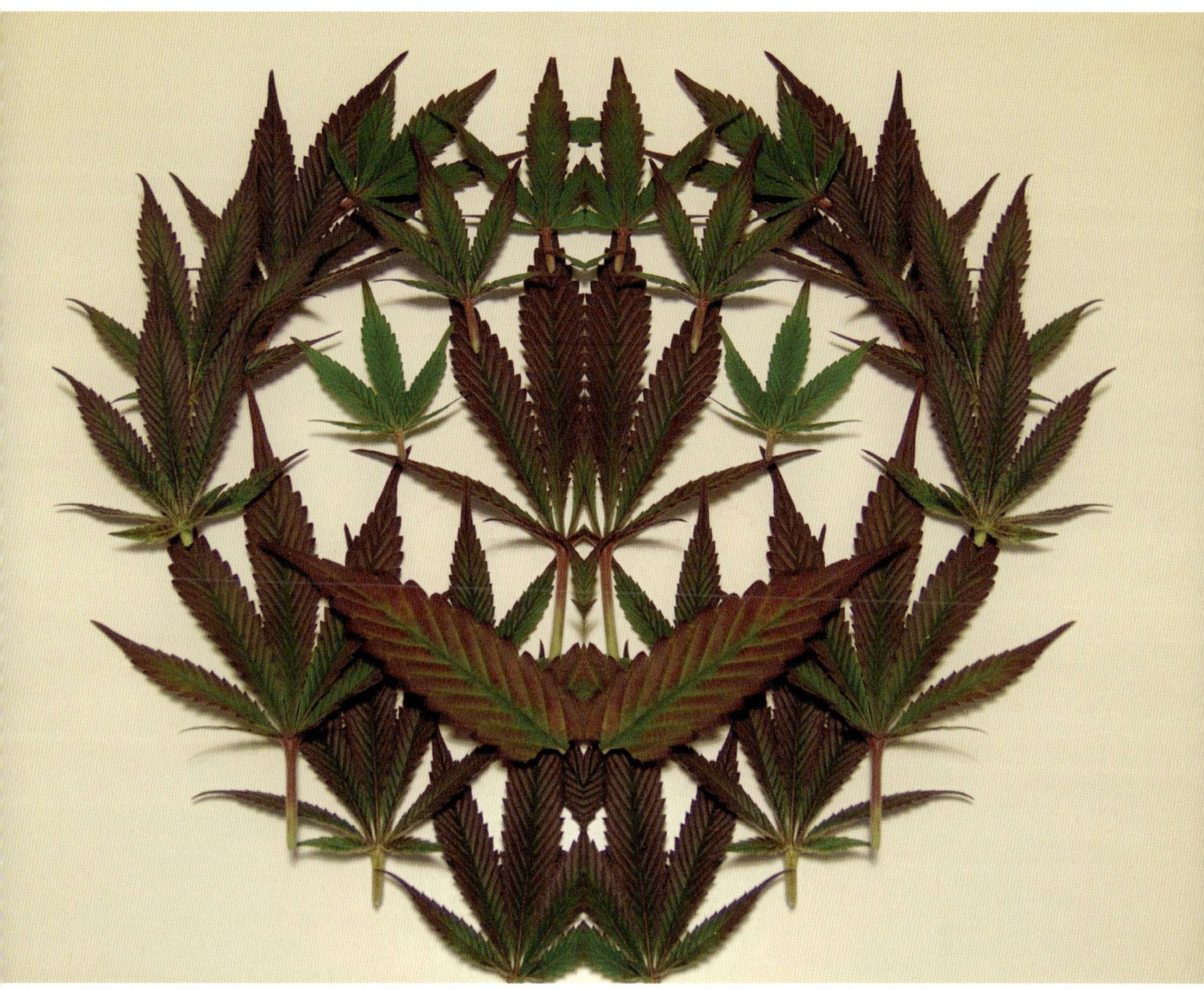

Light and Shadow

previous page—I illuminated this bud with a flashlight on the right side and manipulated the light until I had enough shadow to create some contrast. Doing so added a little depth in the center of the image. I think it worked well.

Put on a Happy Face

above—I created half of a smiley face with fresh-cut leaves from an indica cross and mirrored it. I love the colors here. The image makes me smile every time I see it.

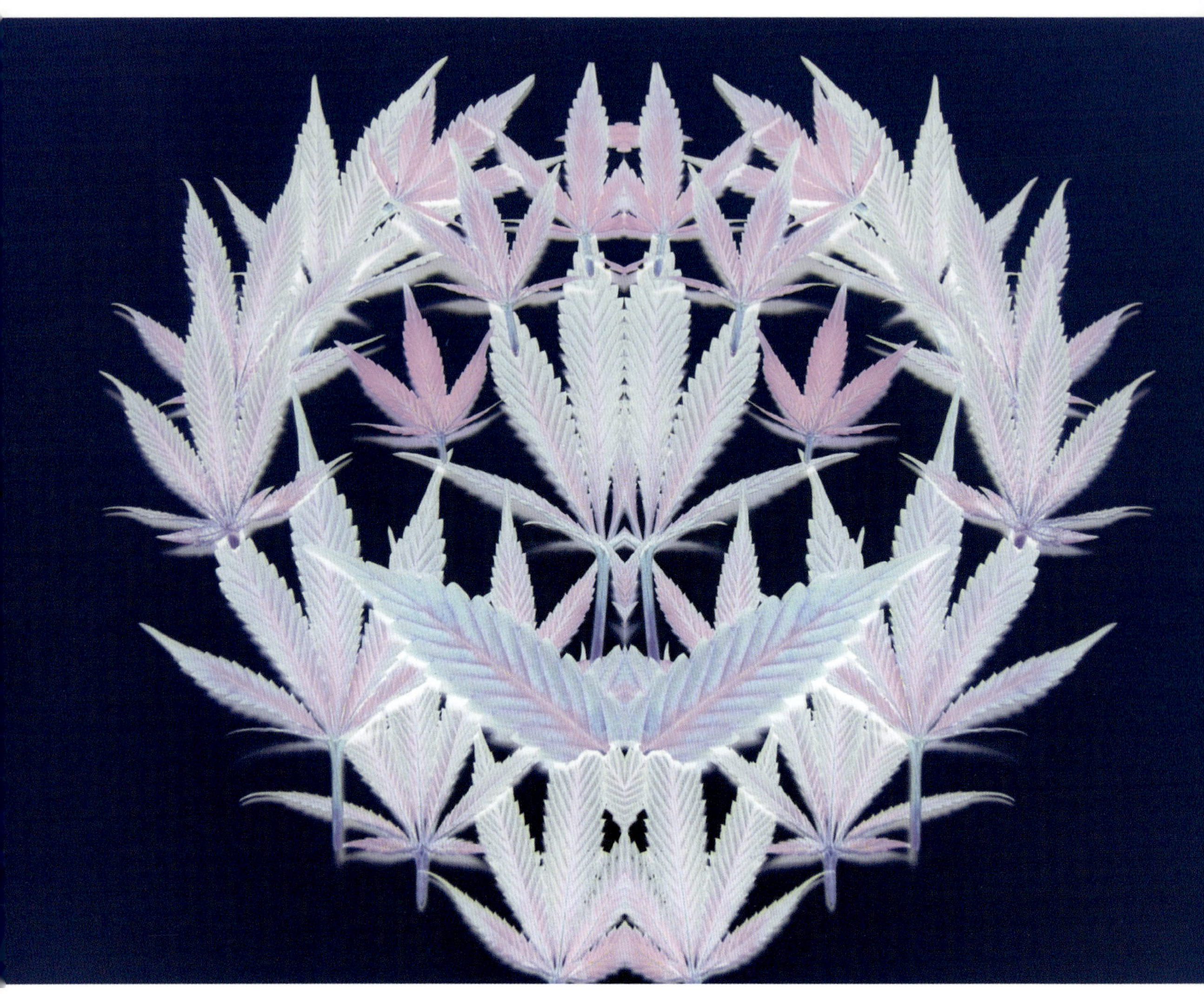

Take Two

above—Here is the same shot shown on the previous page—this time, with a solarized twist. It really pops!

Let the Flames Begin!

following page—Here, I used mylar behind the subject to create reflections that really enhanced the image.

To me, this one looks like several levels of viewing rooms for a stadium overlooking a very shiny floor. The stadium master, in his outrageous canna-costume, announces the beginning of the canna-games, in which only the best buds compete.

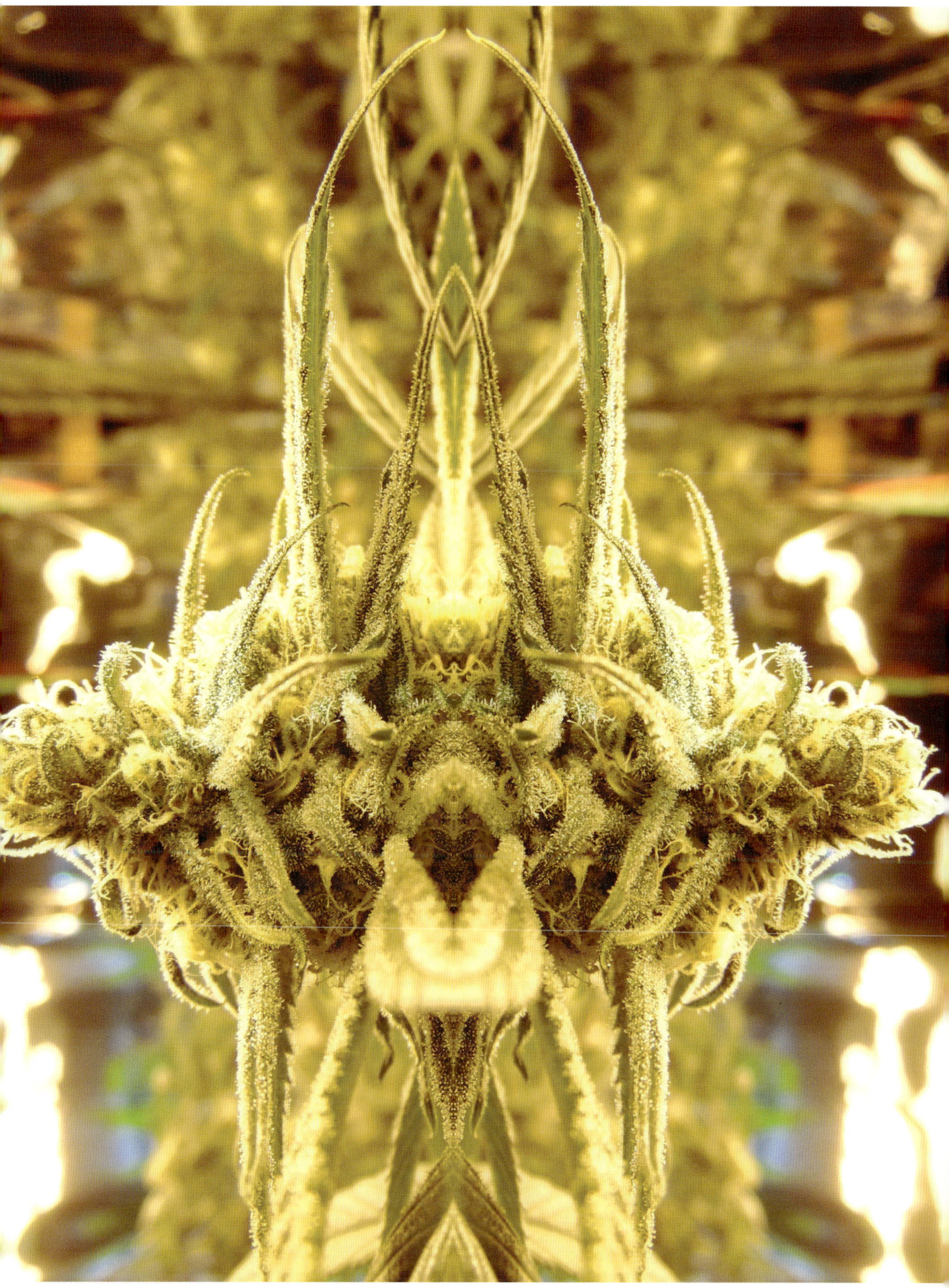

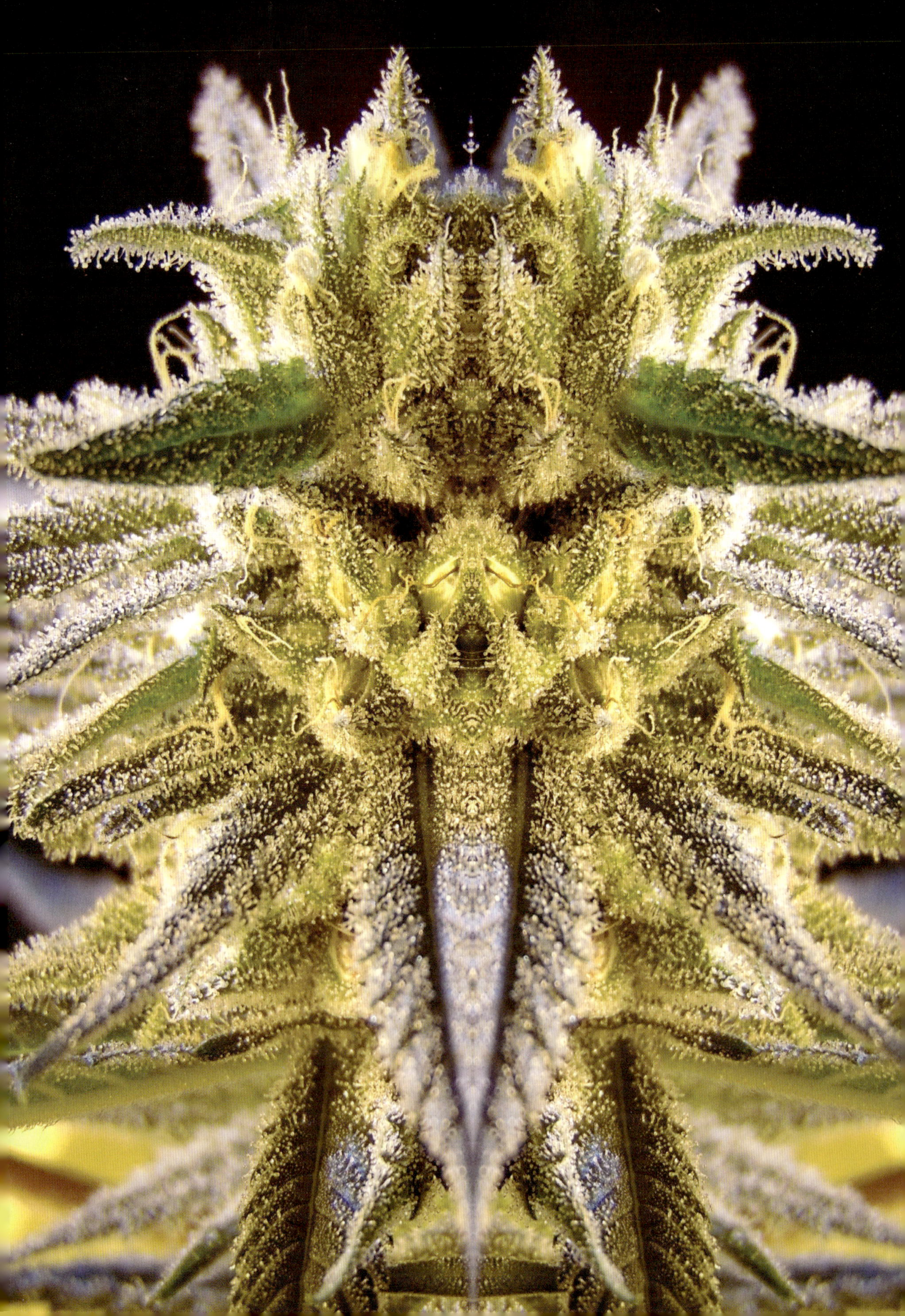

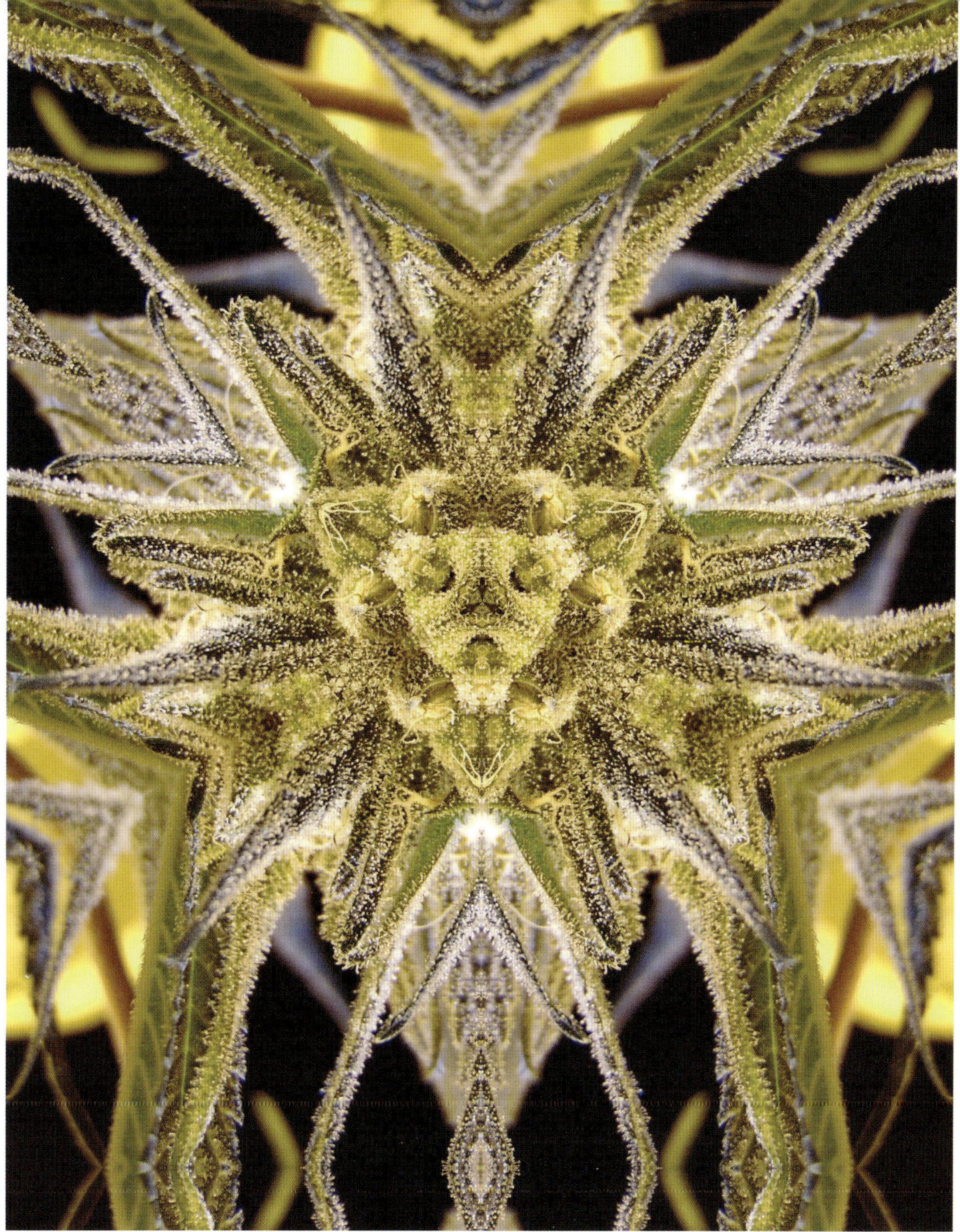

The Space Force

previous page and above—The two images on this page spread show the origins of my own Space Force! On the previous page, you can see my Canna-Dog Combo Unit, also known as CDC-2. Just kidding—it's actually a canna-dog giving another one a piggyback ride.

To create the photograph above, I started with the image on the previous page and created a three-petal kaleidoscope. The orange moon and bird representations at the top of the frame add a nice element to the image.

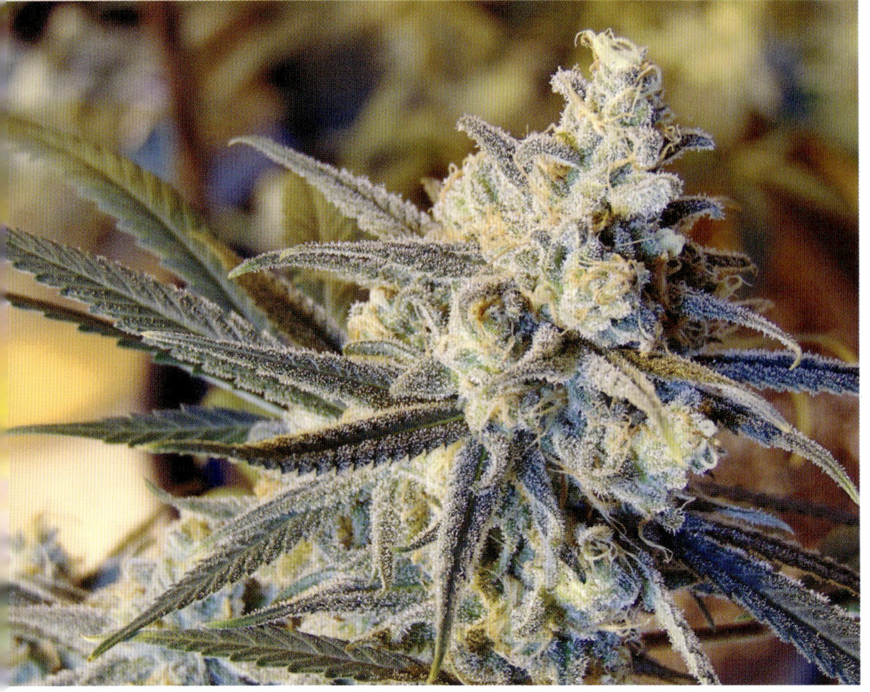

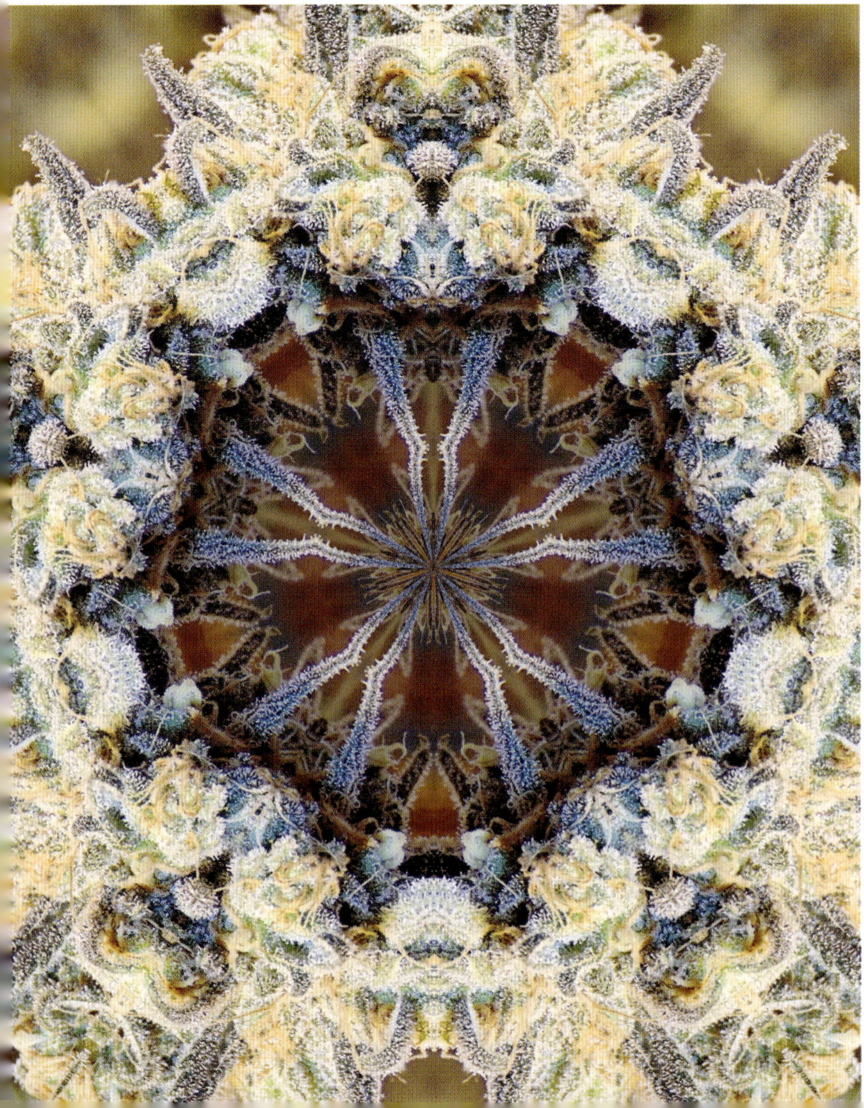

Before and
After

top—She's a beautiful model, isn't she? I love the lighting. Let's see what I can do with this one.

bottom—The image above turned into a five-petal kaleidoscope here. A gateway to an unknown space is created, surrounded by electric pistils. Enter the realm of imagination maximus!

What Do
You See?

following page, top—This is one of those images that can surprise you. What you see from a distance is far different from what you see close-up. Up close, start at the top or bottom and work your way to the center. See how many faces you can pick out. Remember, they don't have to be human faces—most of the time, they aren't.

following page, bottom—Here is the same image shown at the top of the page, flipped 180 degrees. I love it when making a simple change produces a whole new look. To me, the subject looks like a being with a large, blue headdress that extends to a mask.

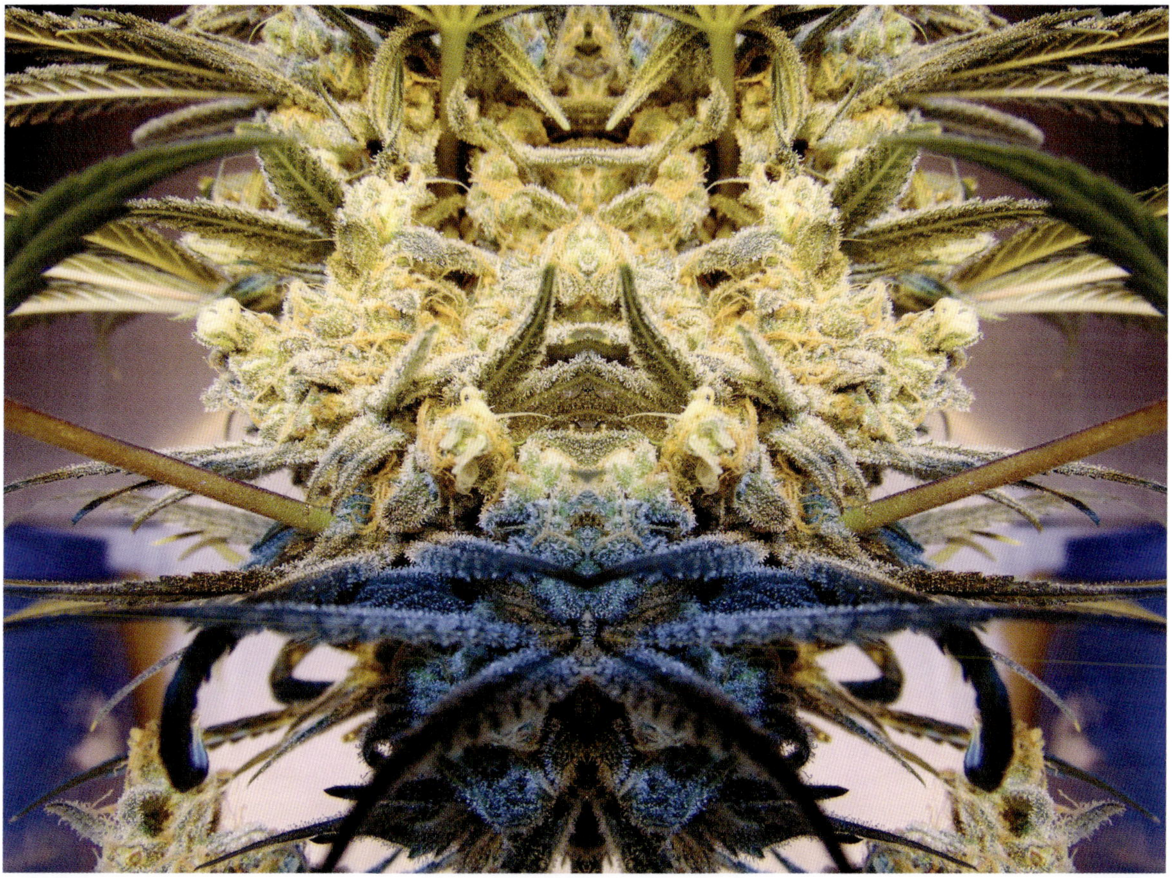

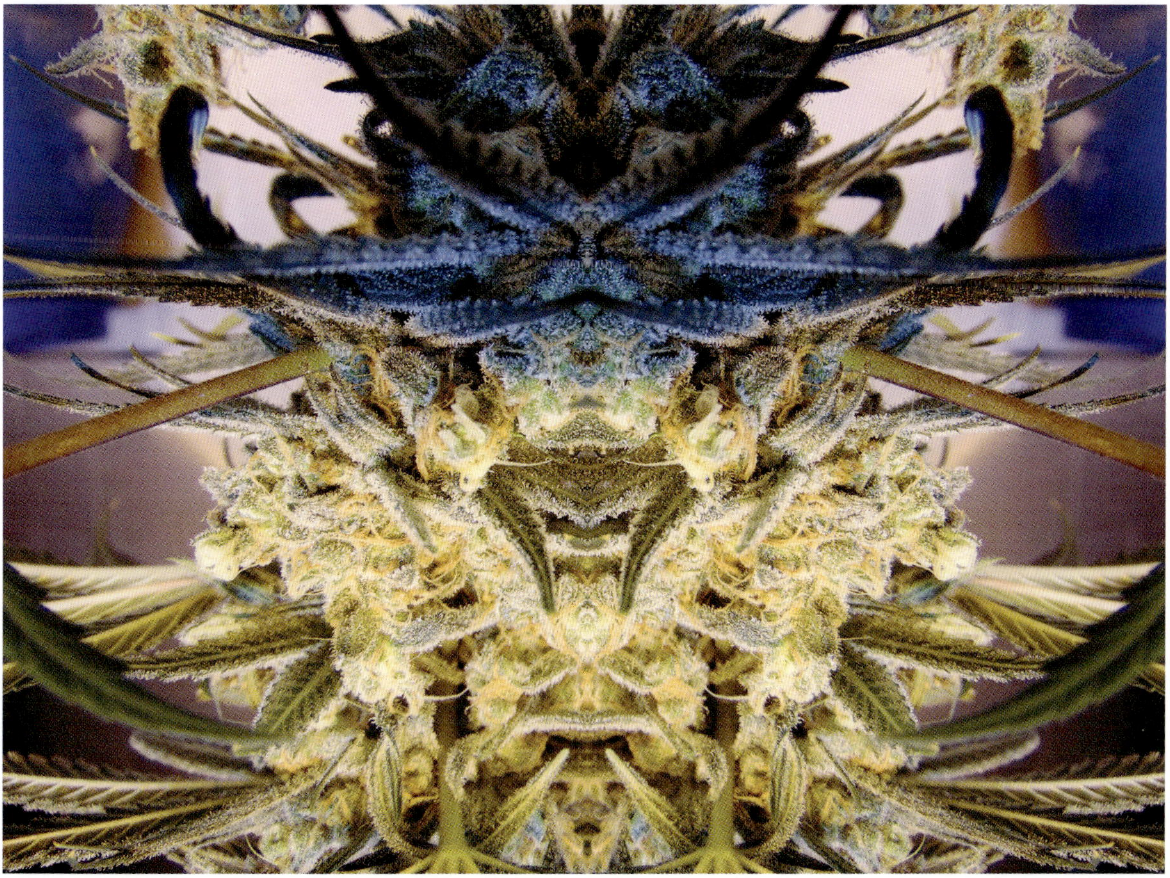

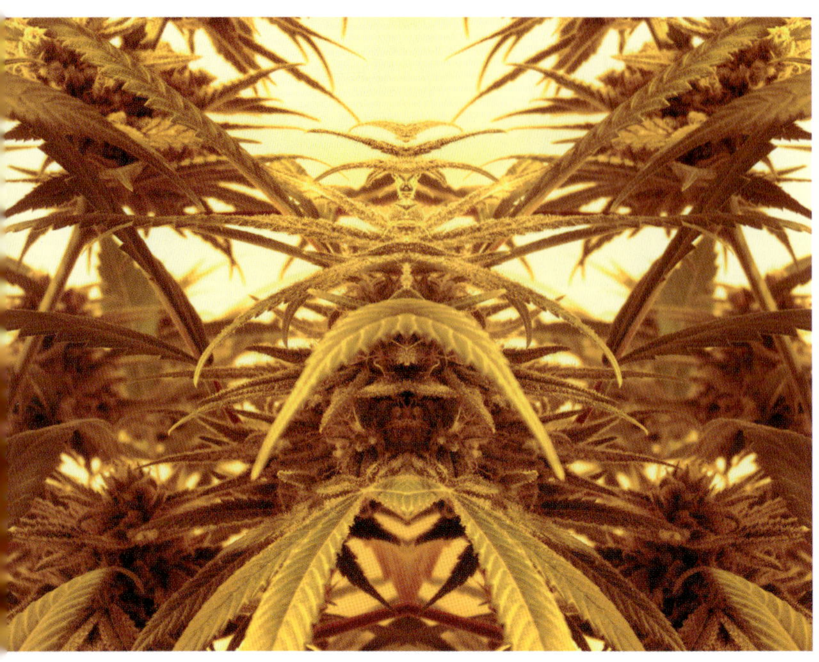

Light It Up

top—The HPS light in the background created a nice effect in this image. We see more canna-birds, a few faces, and some really nice buds.

Front and Back

bottom—I love the way the blurred background plays against the foreground. There's enough of the foreground covering the back to make it easy on the eyes.

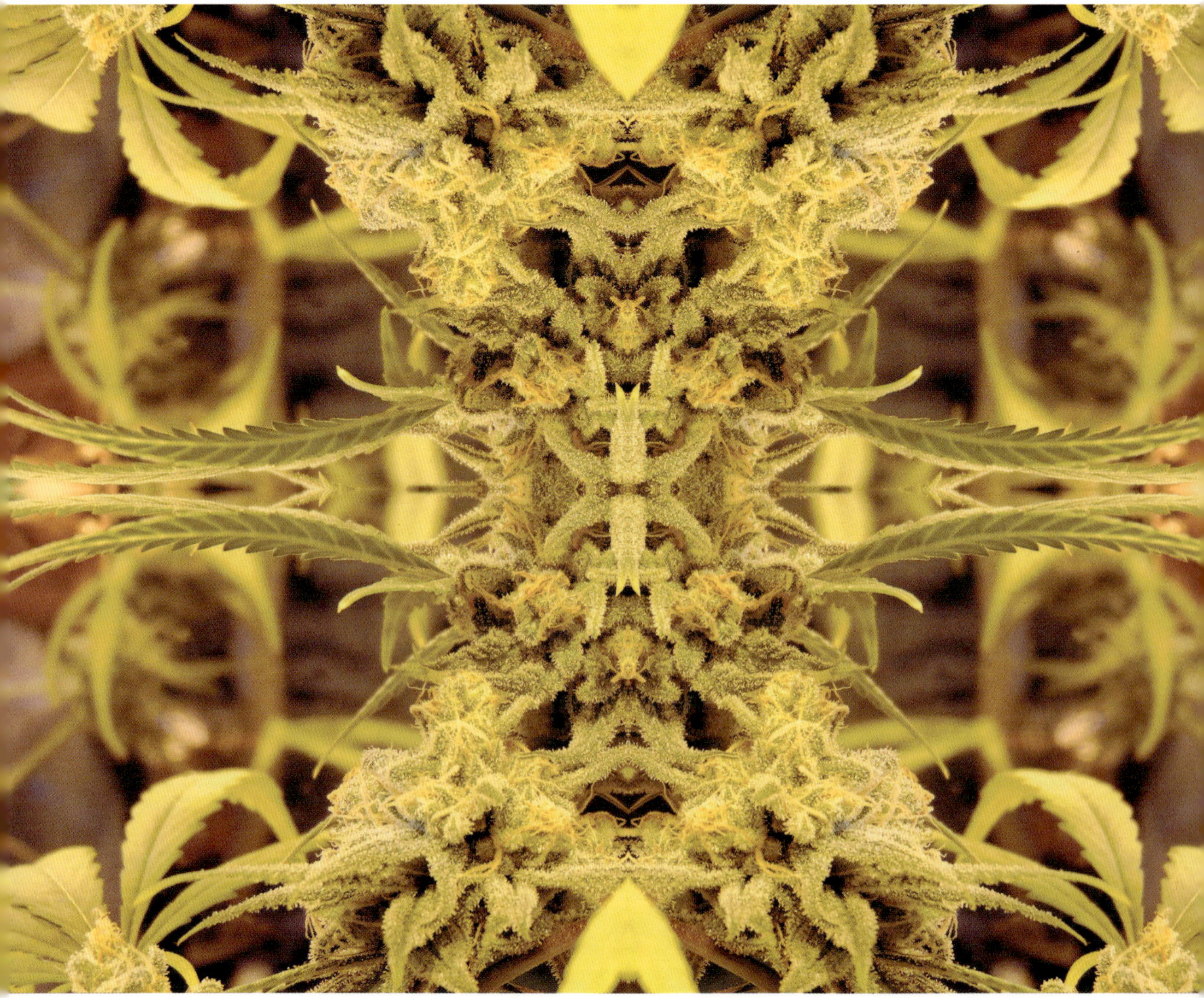

It Takes Two

below—My friend painted this canvas and let me use it for a backdrop for some of his cut buds. I think I was able to make an interesting creature that complements the canvas.

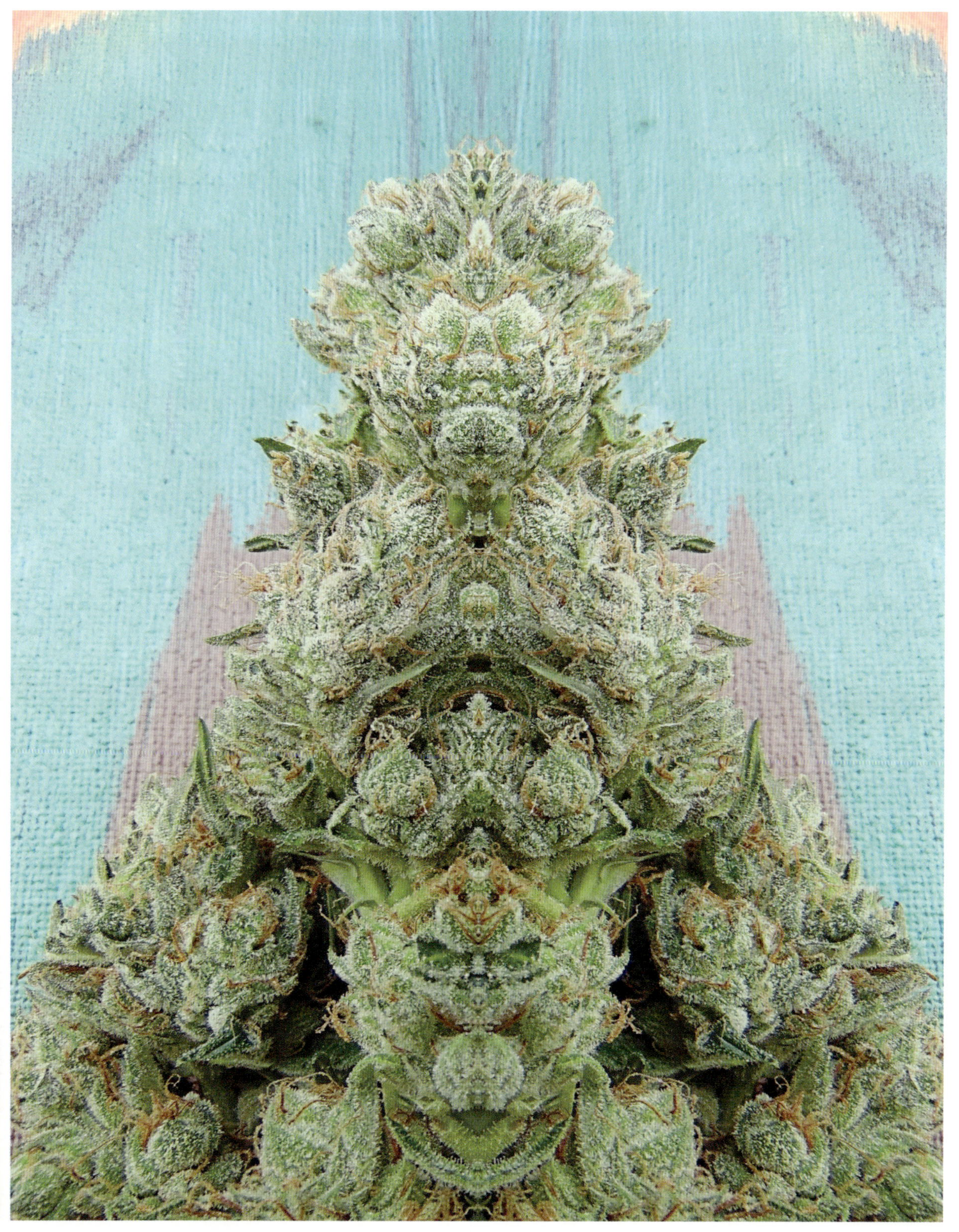

Totem

below—Top to bottom, this plant totem is full of characters. The plant is Blue Dream, of course—and it's in the grow room. The mylar background is full of accentuating leaves and stems.

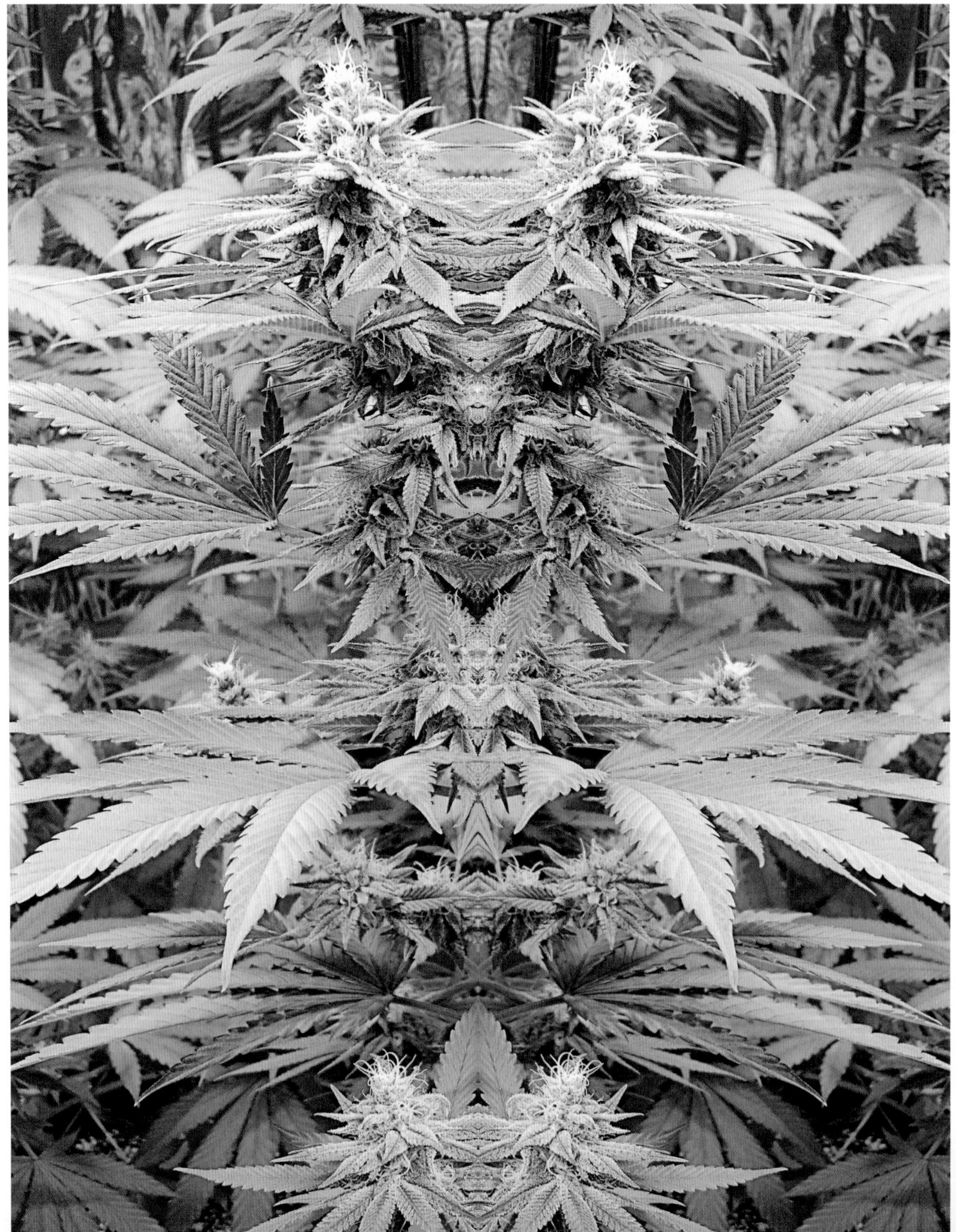

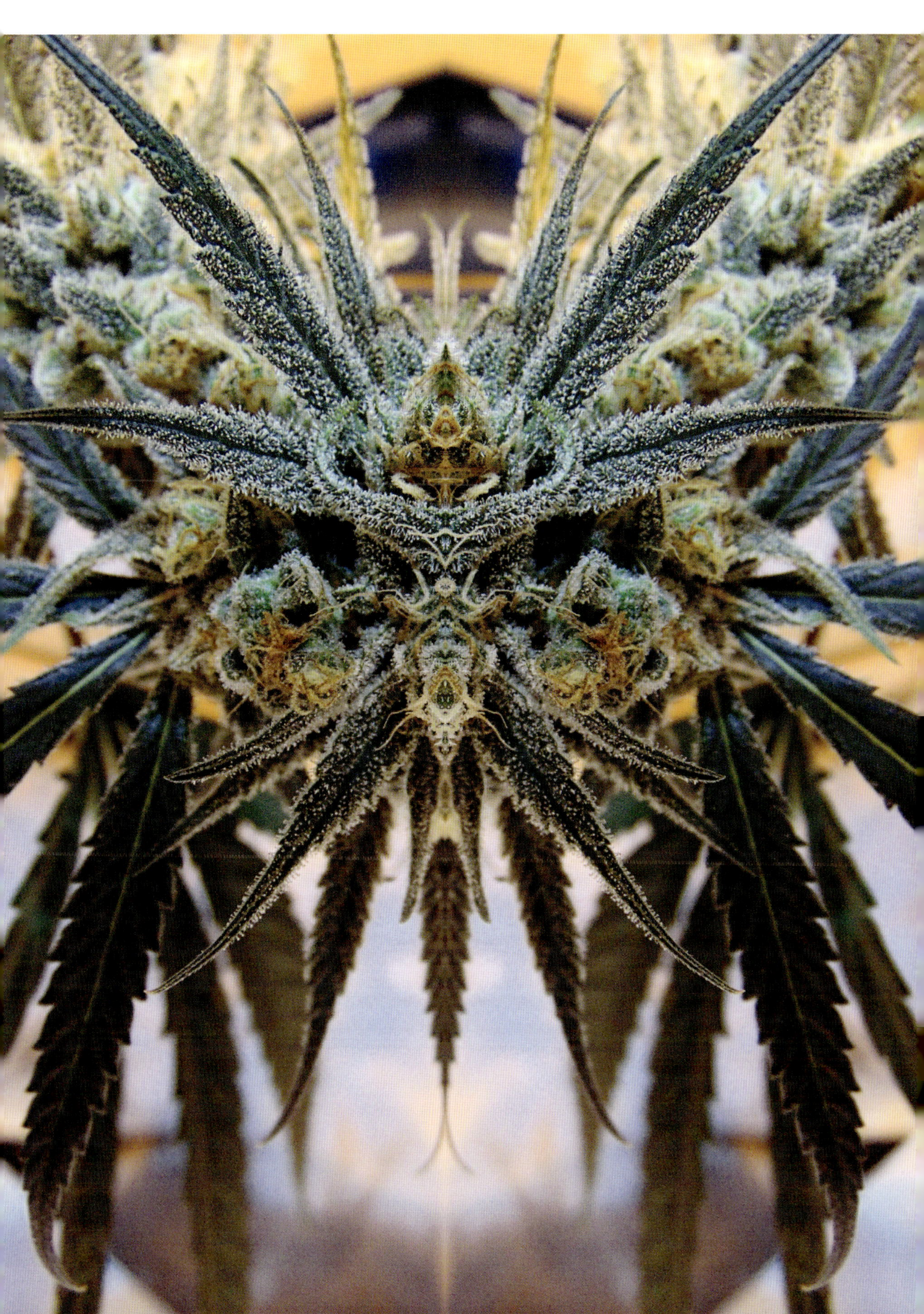

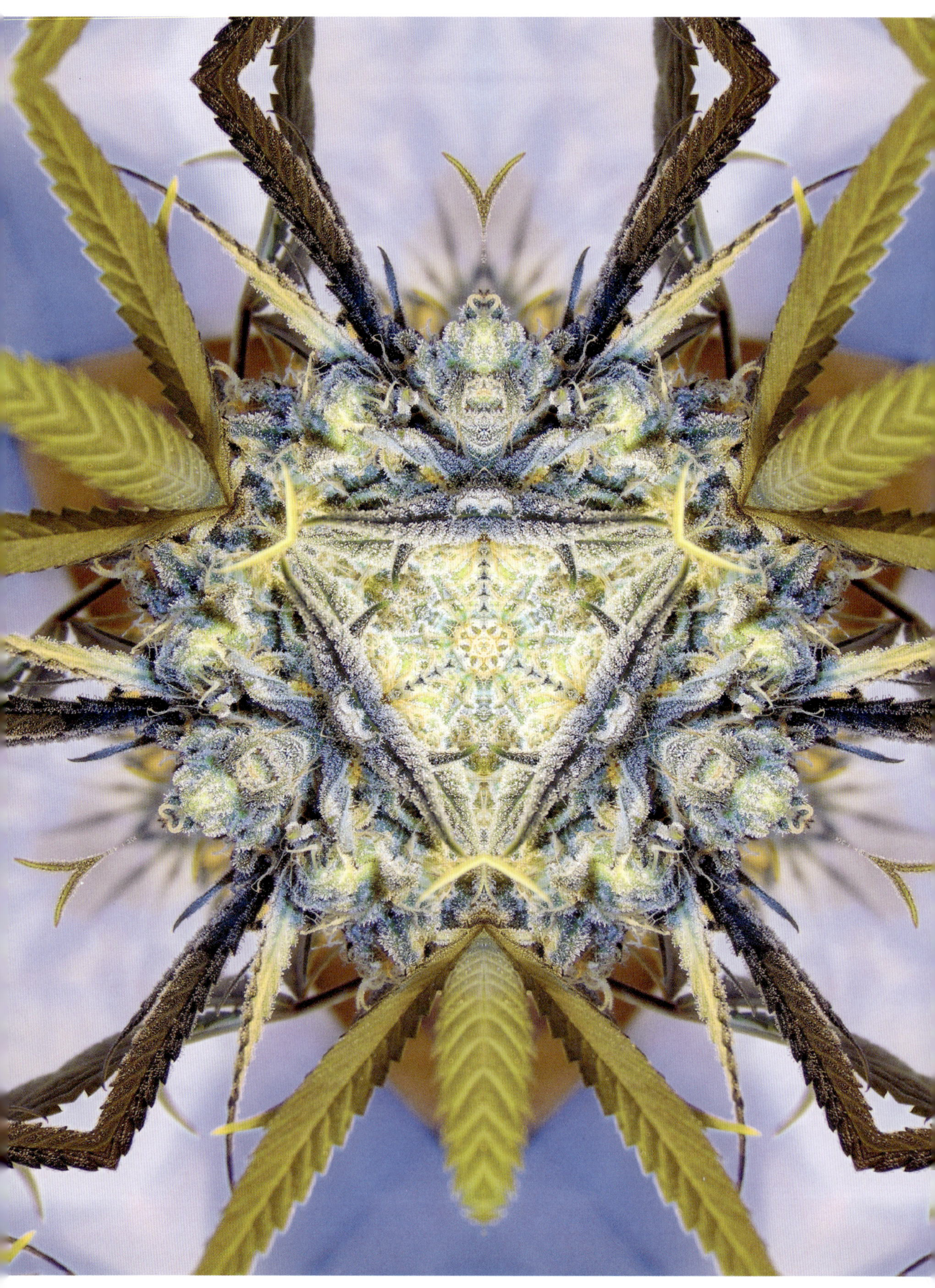

Peace Out

below—This is a mirrored image with a few good faces and beings in it. I like the monkey-like being that photo-bombed me at the top and the weird creature in the center who's flashing two peace signs. I also used this image to create the three-petal portal on the previous page.

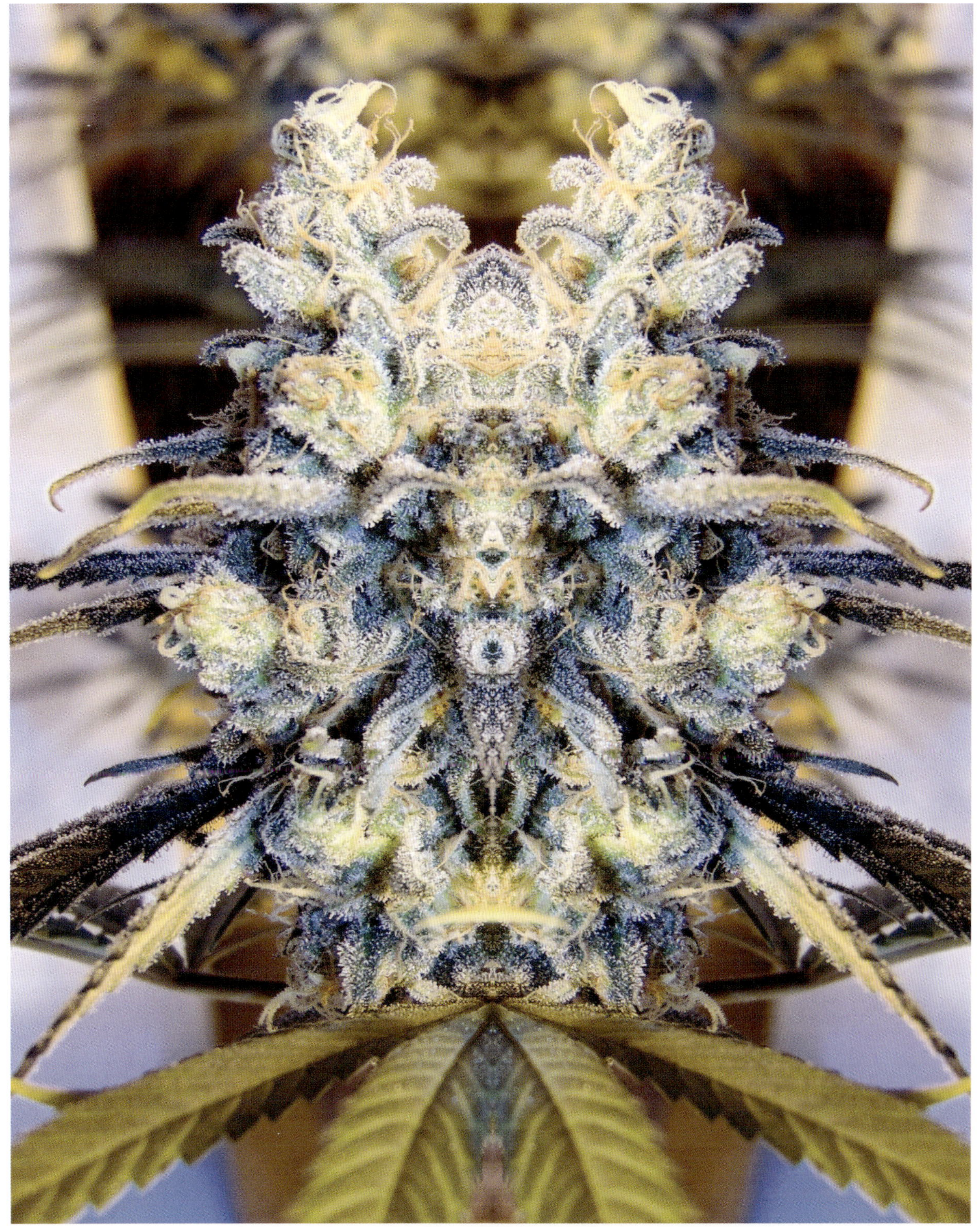

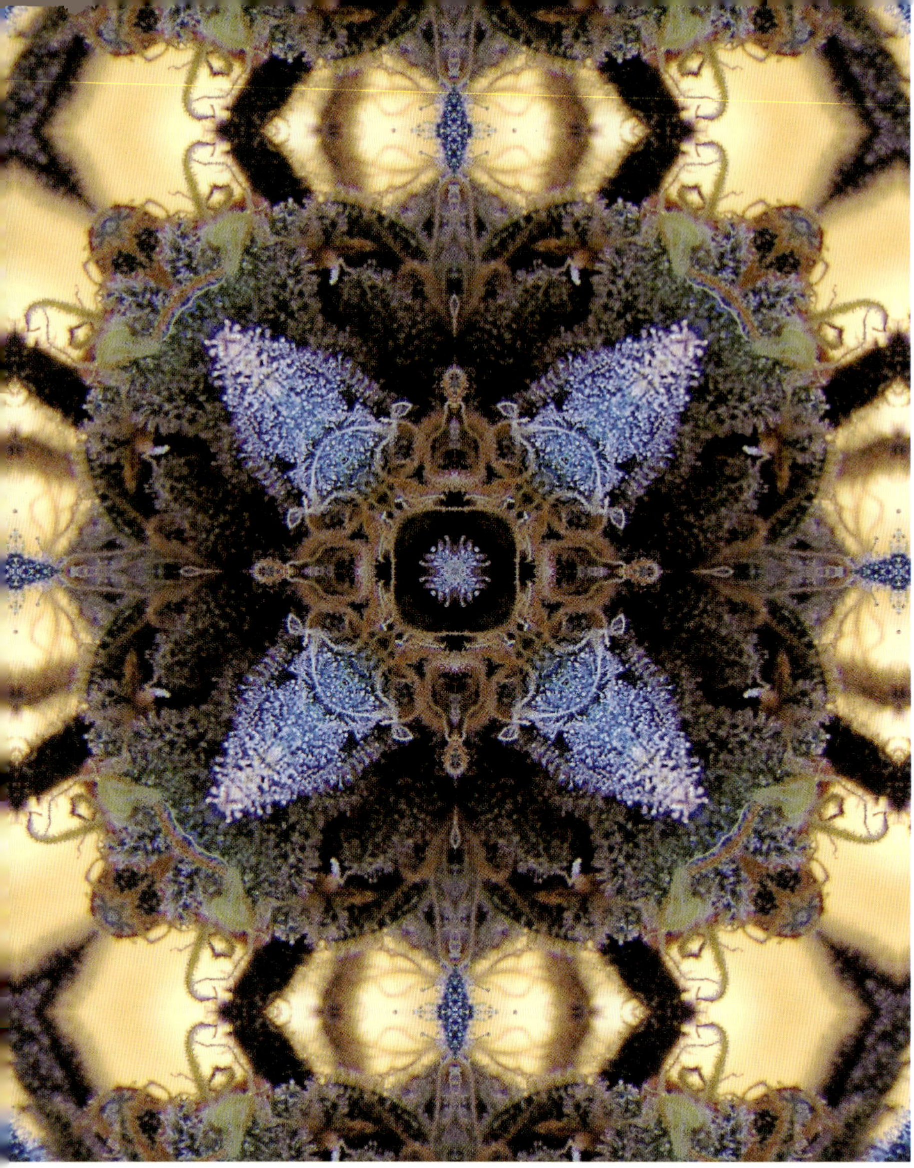

Mandalas

top—Creating kaleidoscope images is fun. Here, the pistils are just starting to recede, bending at the tips and forming fine detail that draws the eye inward. The way the light ignites the trichomes, giving the impression of a blue flame from a torch, is just beautiful.

bottom—So many petal options make for a wide variety of possibilities to alter an image. This image, and the one above it, remind me of intricate stained glass windows. I love the way they came together in the form of mandalas, and the colors are amazing.

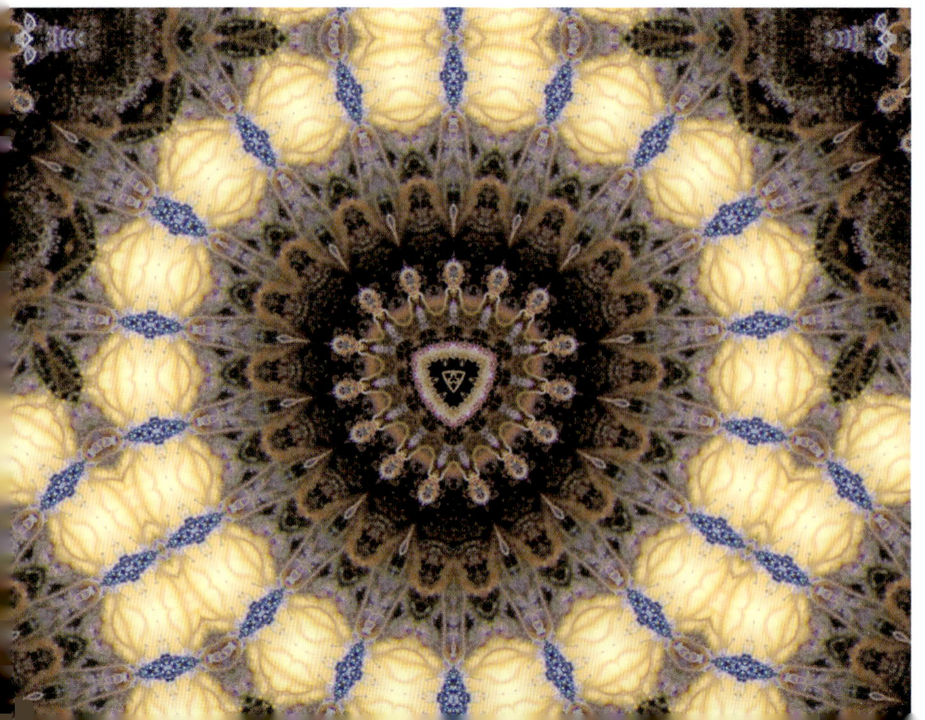

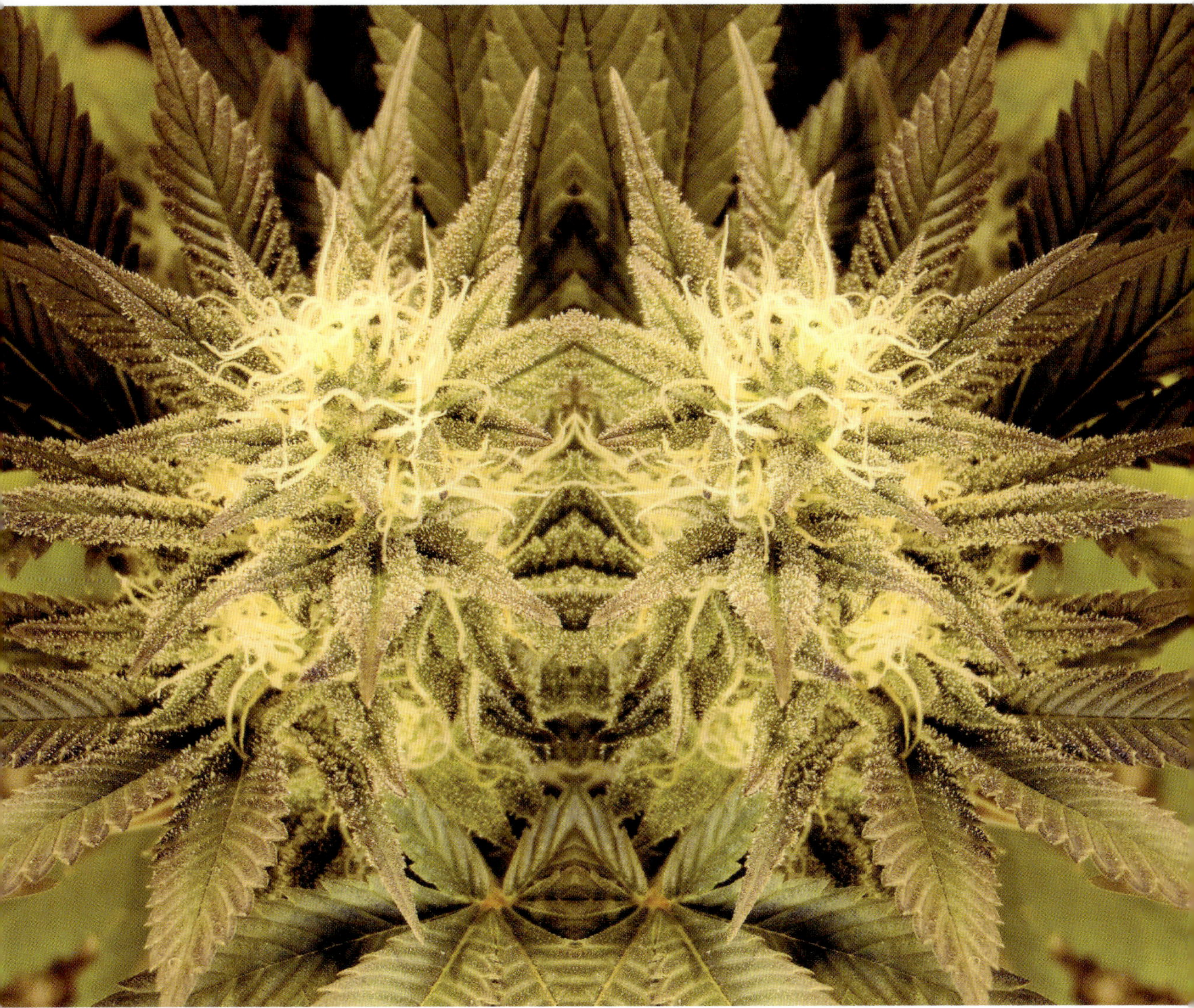

Canna-Buddha

above—Our bud, canna-Buddha. His wisdom is a great match for the healing qualities of cannabis. In this image, he relaxes on his indica pillow and breathes in the earthy scents. He thinks to himself, "The mind is everything. What you think, you become. Three things cannot be long hidden: the sun, moon, and the truth. We are shaped by our thoughts. When the mind is pure, joy follows like a shadow that never leaves."

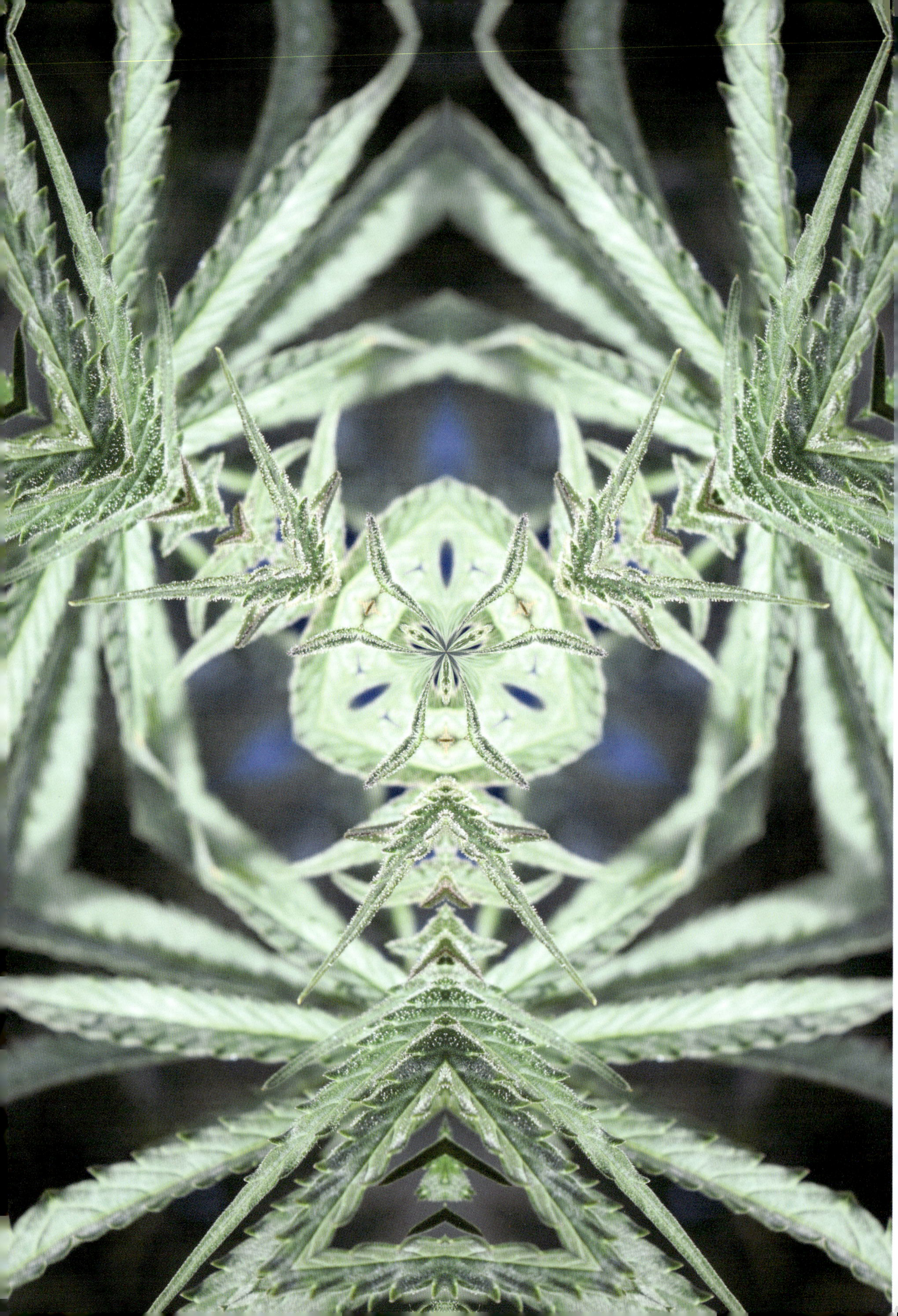

Many Shades of Green

previous page—Leaf play.

below—This mirrored image was made with numerous plants. There may be a record number of beings' faces in this image. I love the mylar effects at the top. Slight wrinkles in the material always make for good reflections.

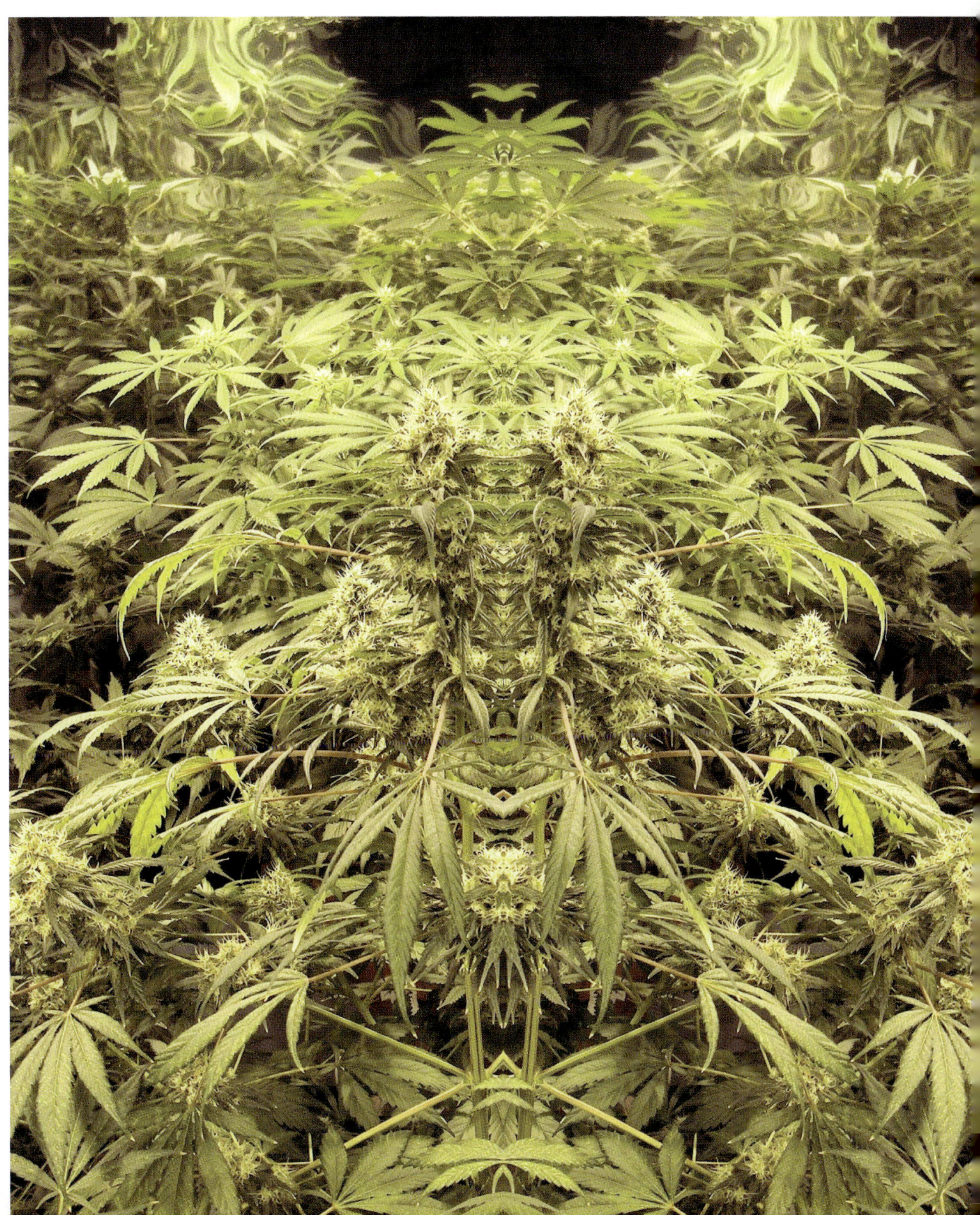

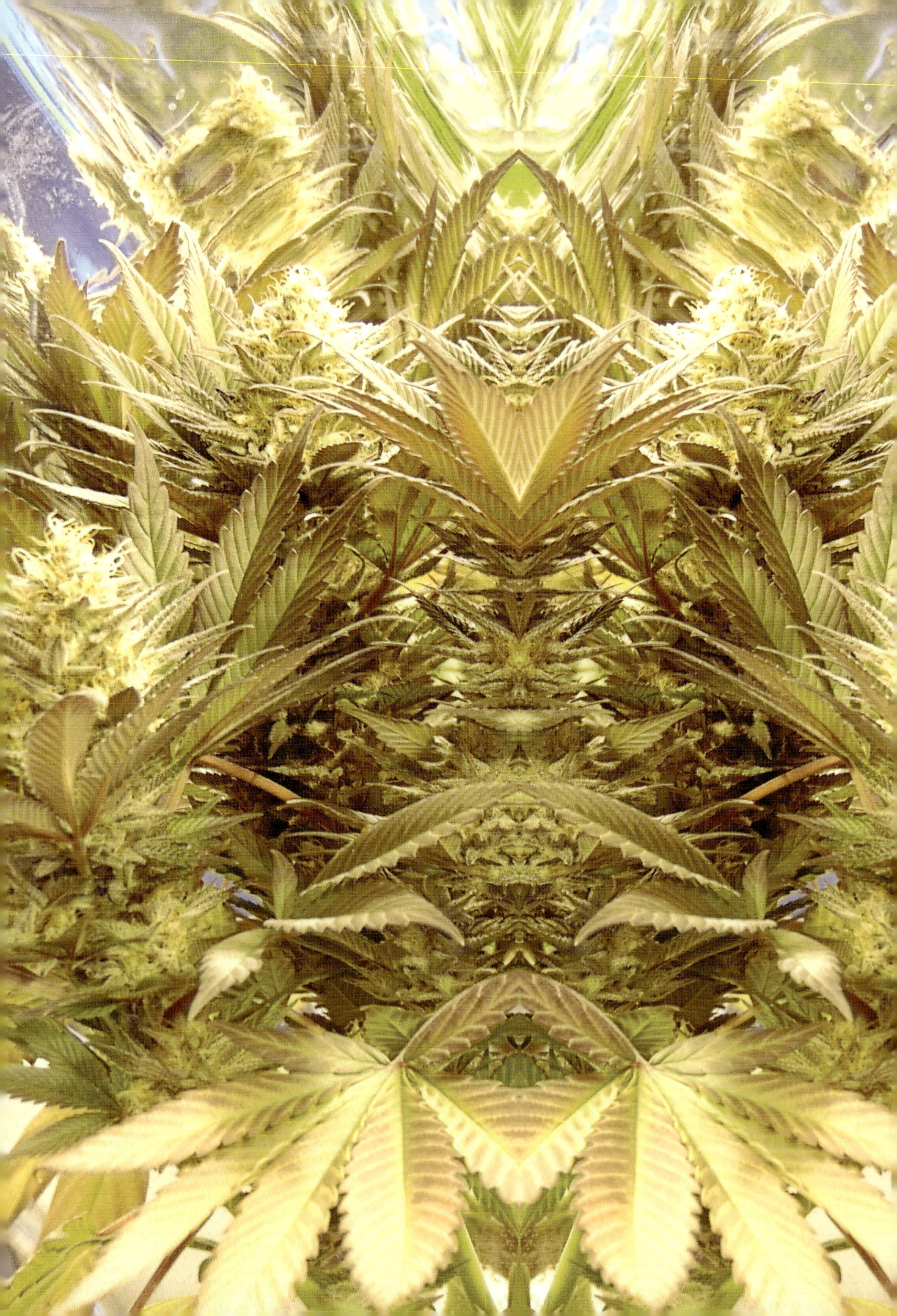

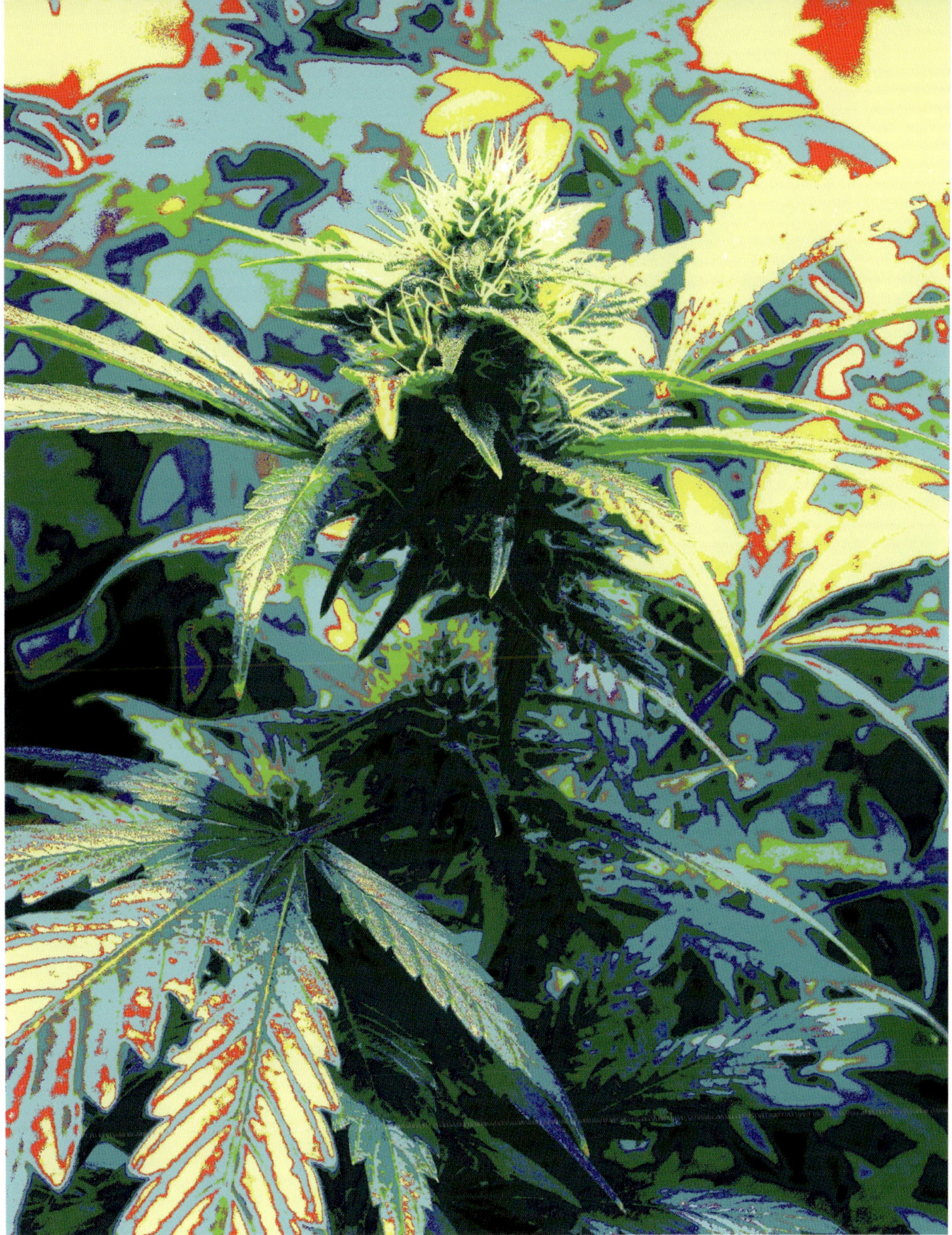

Shades of Anonymous

previous page—I see a representation of Anonymous at the very top, and a bunch of cool beings and faces down the middle.

Just Groovy

above—While playing with the effects in my editing program, I found several interesting options to add a psychedelic look to my images. The following few photos reflect the diversity of creative options available to me.

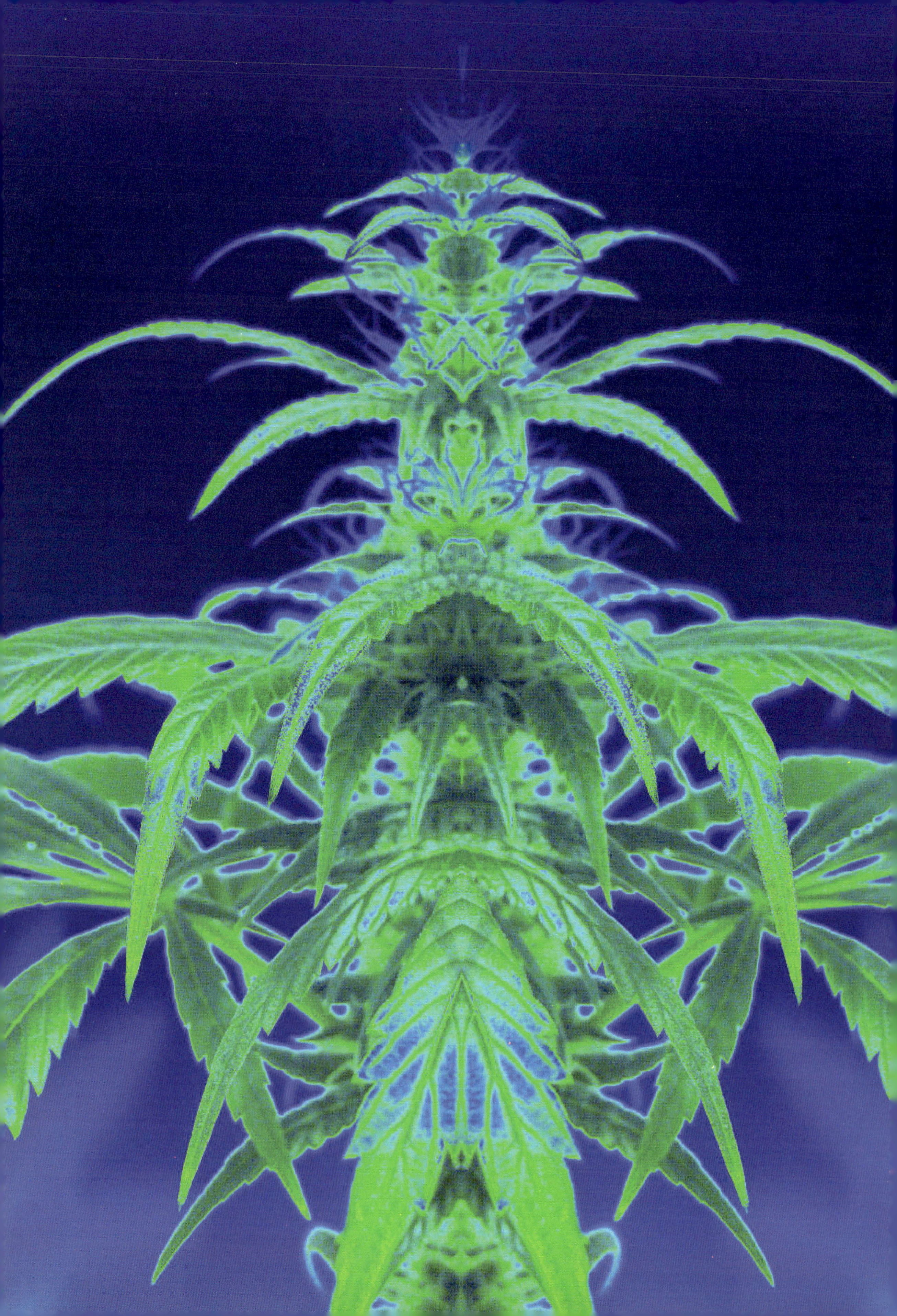

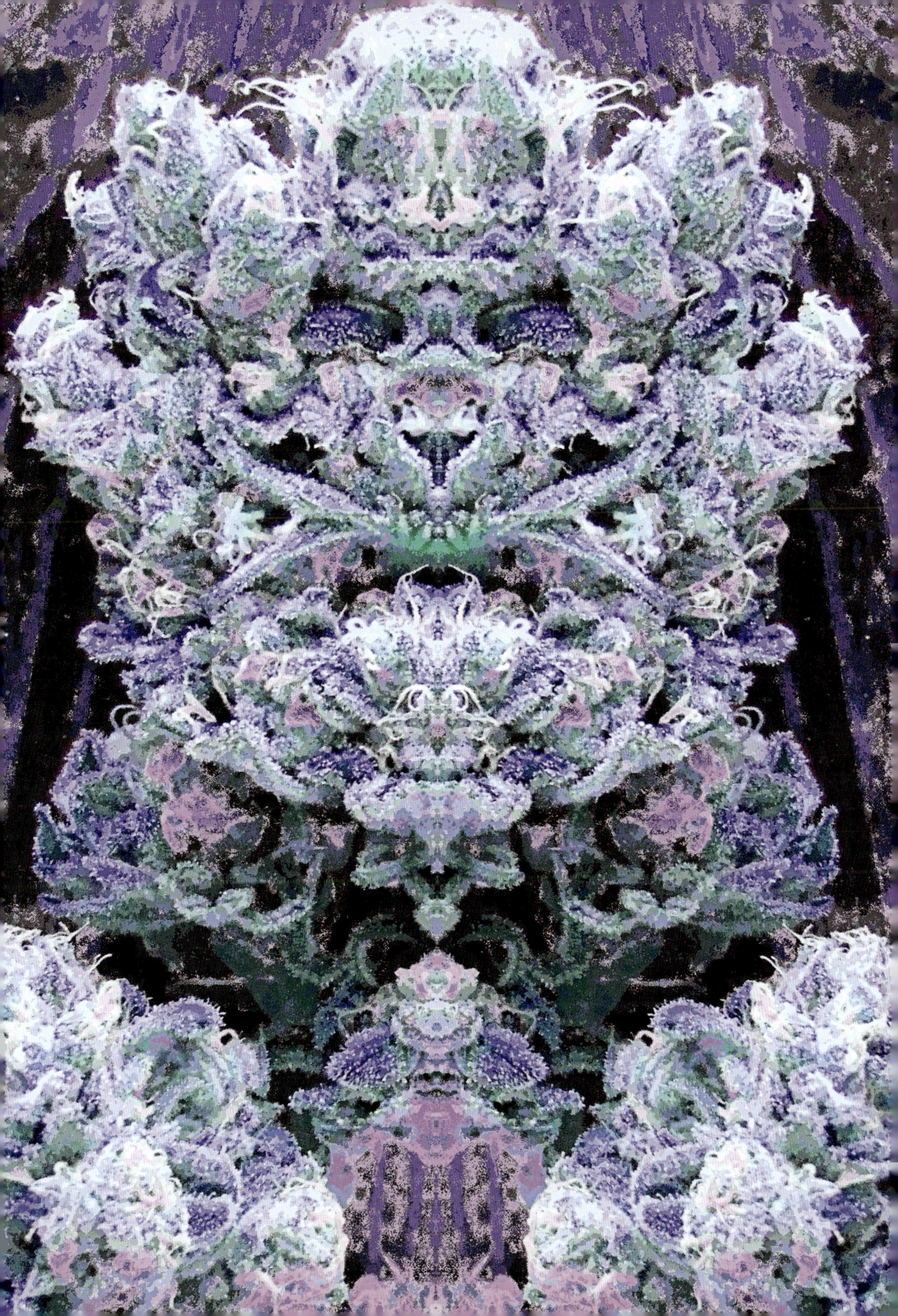

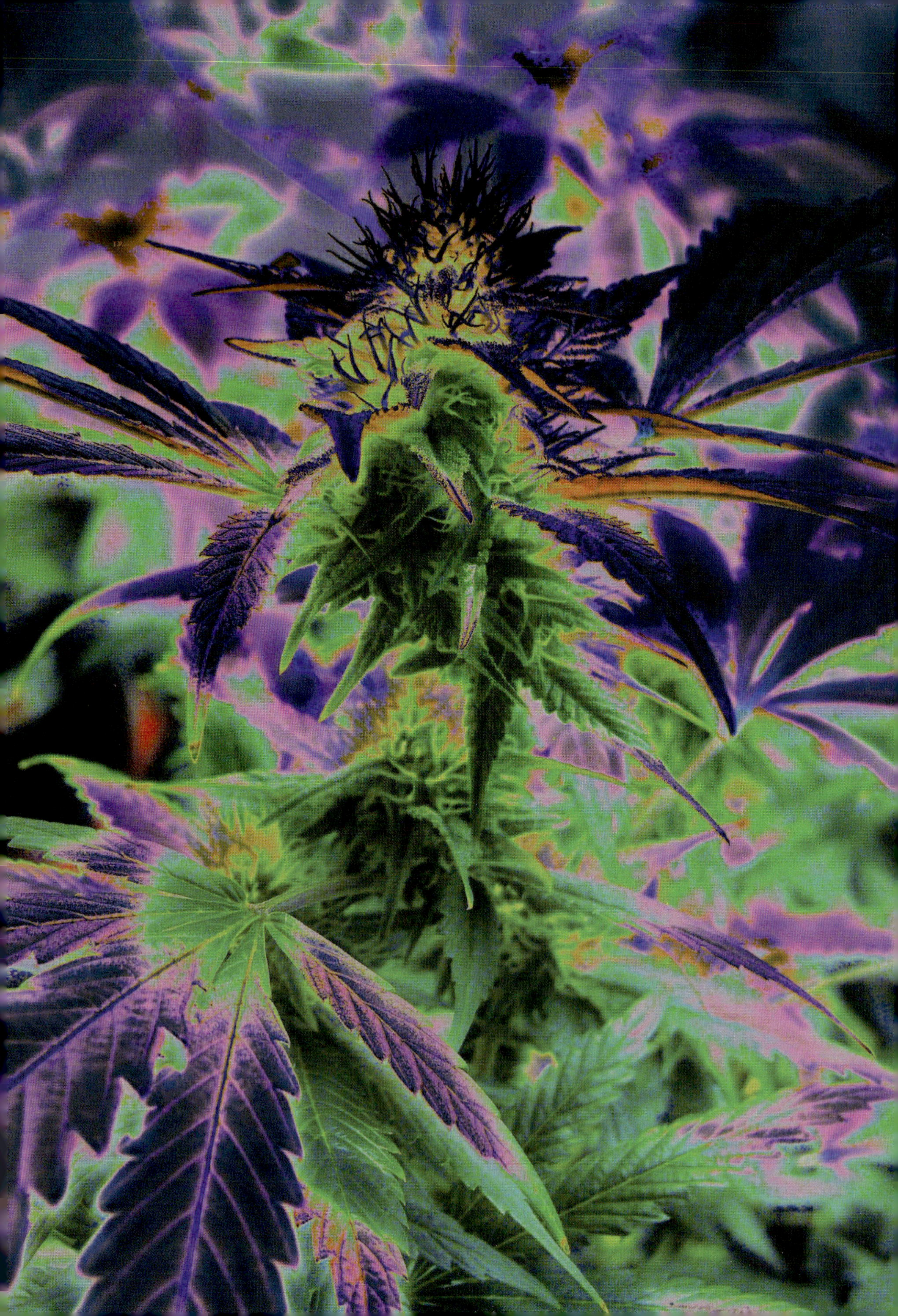

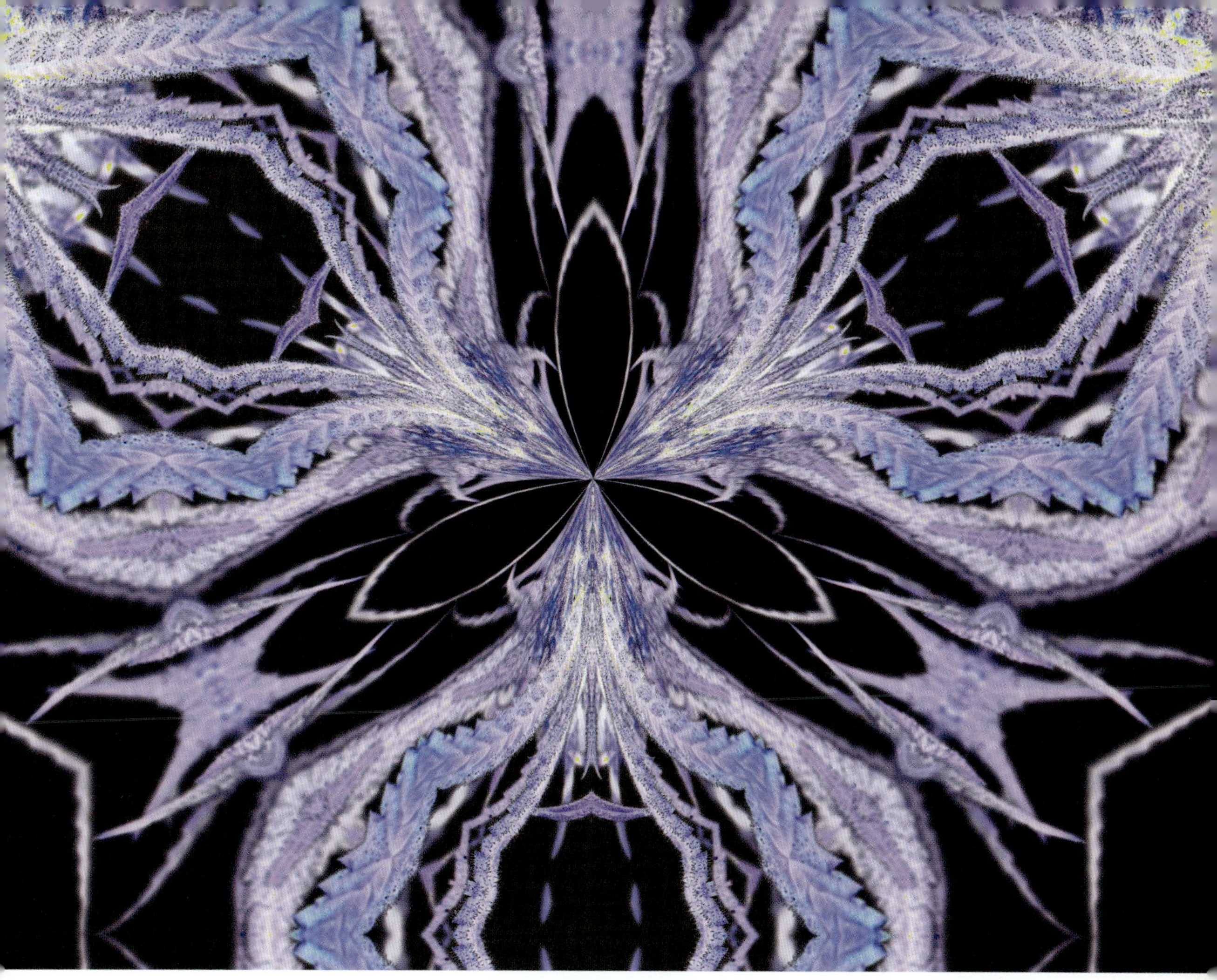

Strange Birds

above—Strange bird-like beings hover over and under a caricature wearing a bow tie in the outer bottom third of the image. He has a big nose! The rest of this three-petal leaf kaleidoscope is just kind of spacey.

Distorted

right—Distorted high-pressure sodium lights set the stage for this odd creation. Strange birds are highlighted in a frame of stalks, and the faces are all happy—especially the one of the dog at the top.

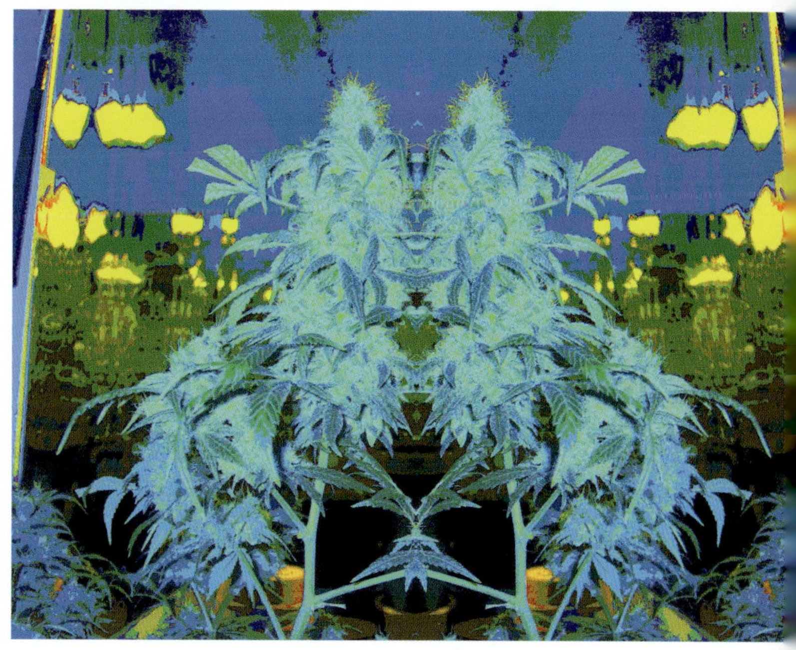

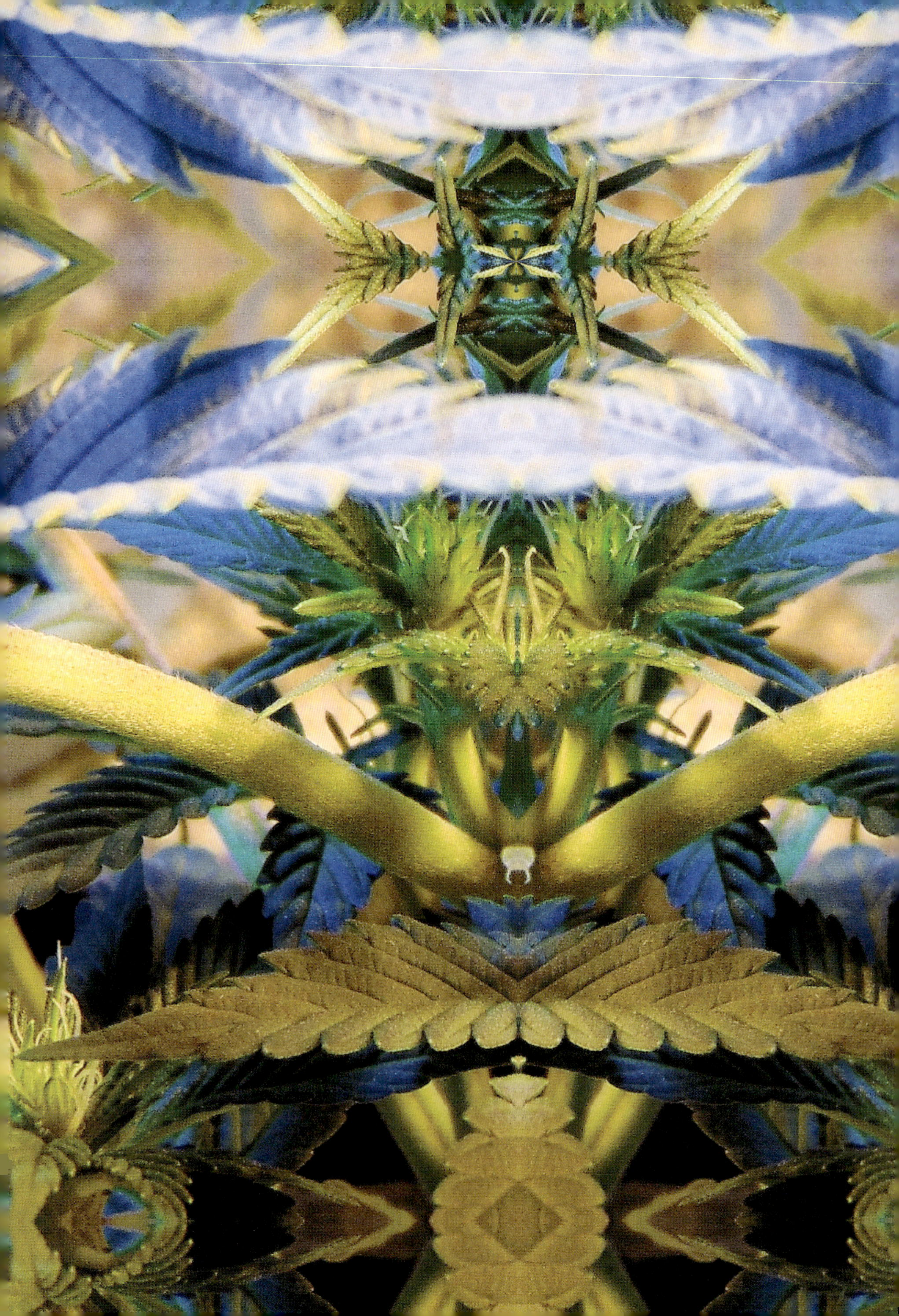

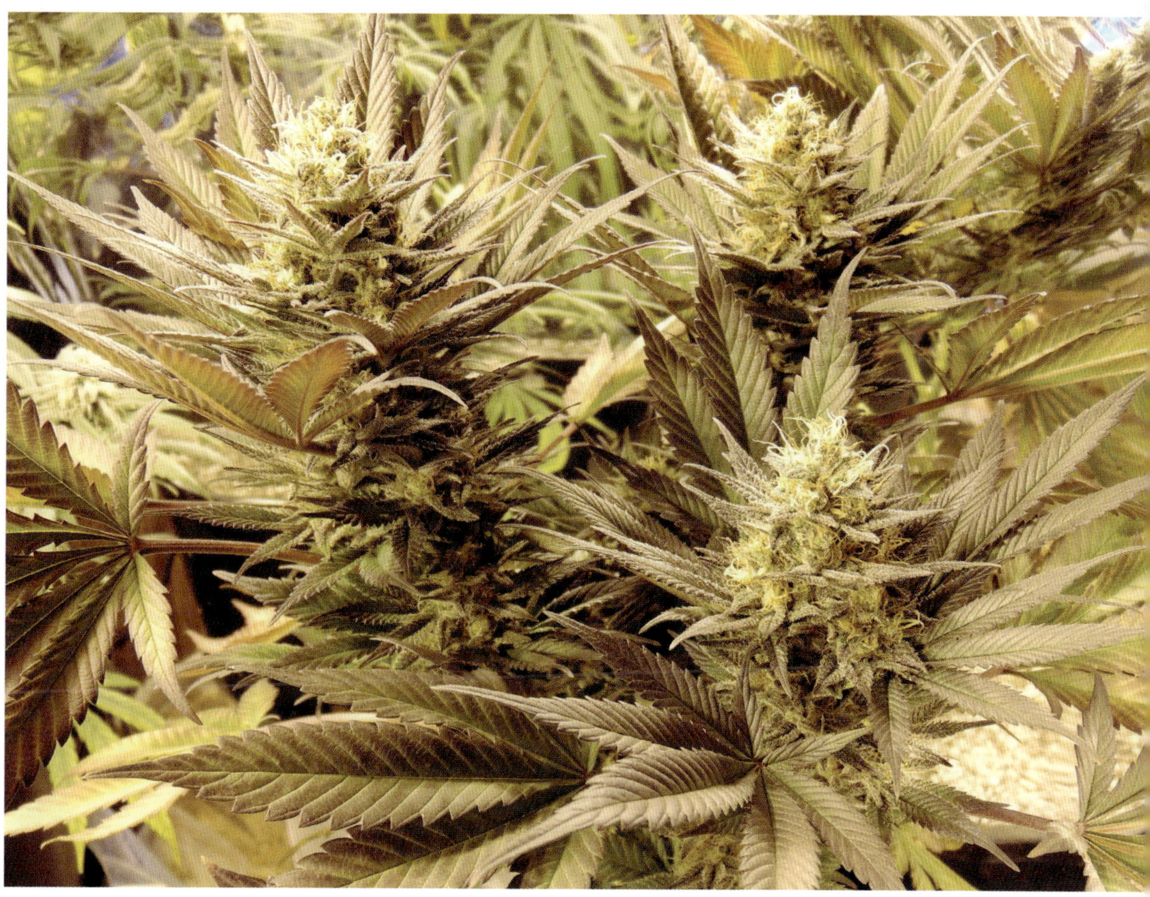

Carnival

left—This young indica had only been flowering for two weeks. That's obvious with the small buds, but how it came out looking like a lady in a Rio Carnival costume, exposing herself to the camera, I will never know.

A Preview

above—I used this image of a maturing indica to create the following two images. She is beautiful but grew too short and only had good buds at the top of the dense canopy. The plant's sisters had hermaphroditic tendencies, and that's not desirable, so the strain had to go. Sometimes it happens like that.

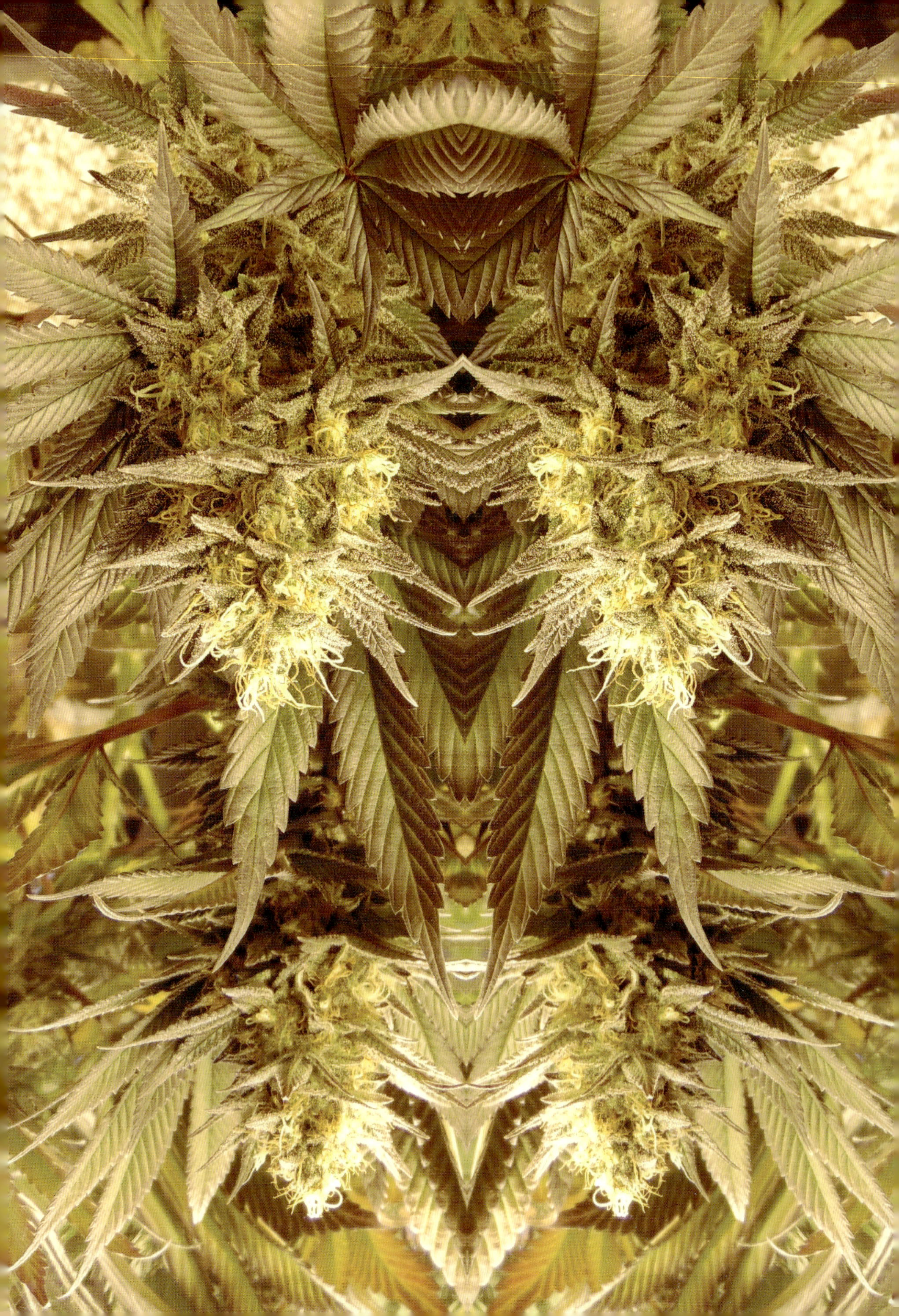

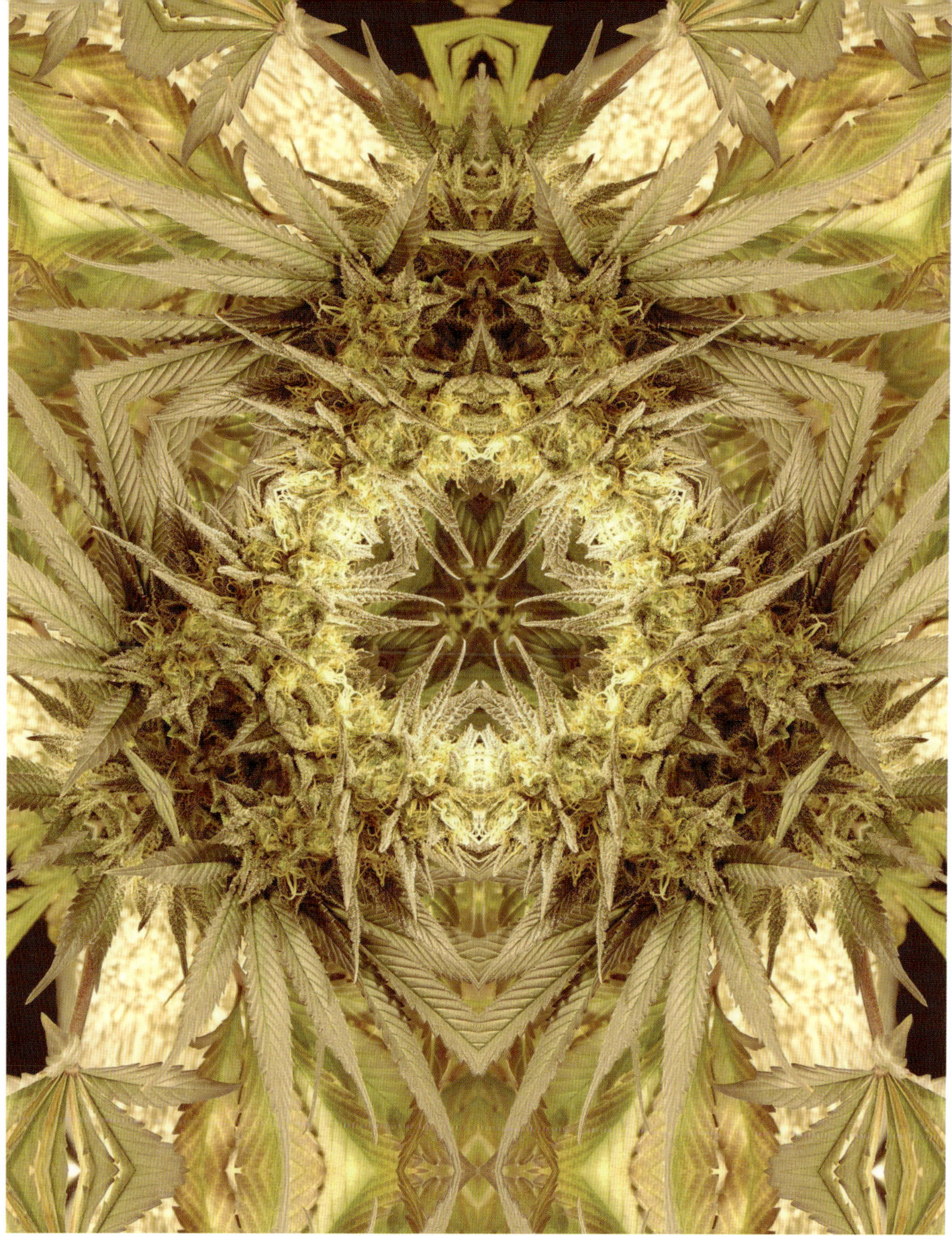

A Curious Combination

previous page—I know it's a little strange to see live buds hanging upside down, and perlite at the top of a picture, but I think this combo makes for an intriguing image.

above—This is a six-petal kaleidoscope made from the image on the previous page. There are two Valkyries (though not so feminine-looking, I must add) at the top and bottom. If you look carefully, you'll see a small, beautiful woman with a little white pendant holding a dude's head; he has wide-open eyes, and his tongue is sticking out.

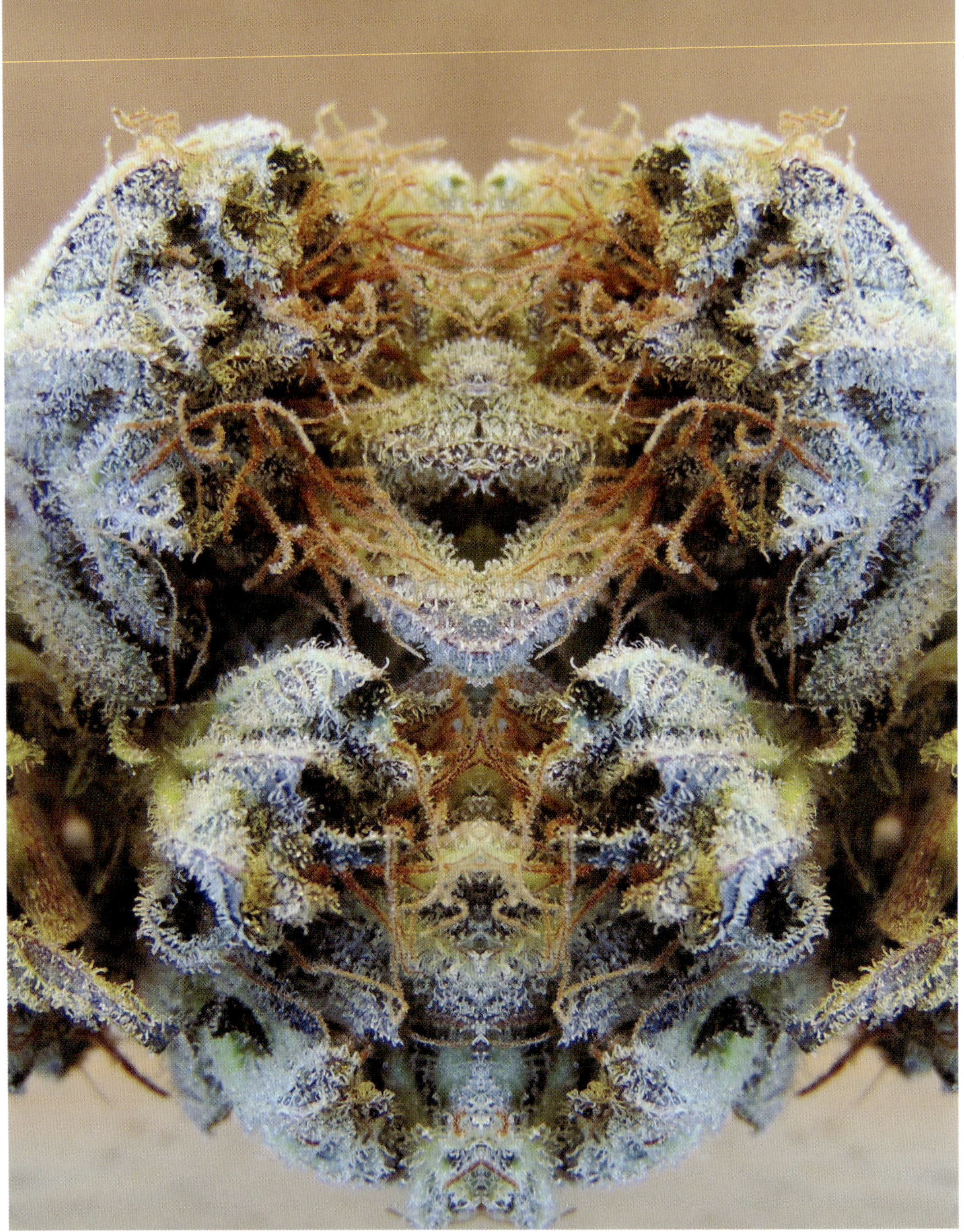

Blue Dream

above—This dry Blue Dream flower, as a whole, looks happy. The big smile near the top tells me this. I look at his trichome-covered hands and see he has captured a person. In the sticky, lovely scented trichomes is Bill Schuette, defeated in his run for governor of Michgan.

See the panic on his face? He is the one who ordered most of the provisioning centers in Michigan to be closed. People paid for the certification, paid the state to process their applications, and then were denied access to their medication. Bye-bye, Schuette!

Pure Power

right—The moment of impact between two equal forces.

Being and Birds

below—See the big lips near the bottom center? The near-vertical nostrils give evidence of the face and head of this being. It has buds for shoulders, stems for arms, and big leaves for hands. Behind that being, the canna-birds fly off into the sunset.

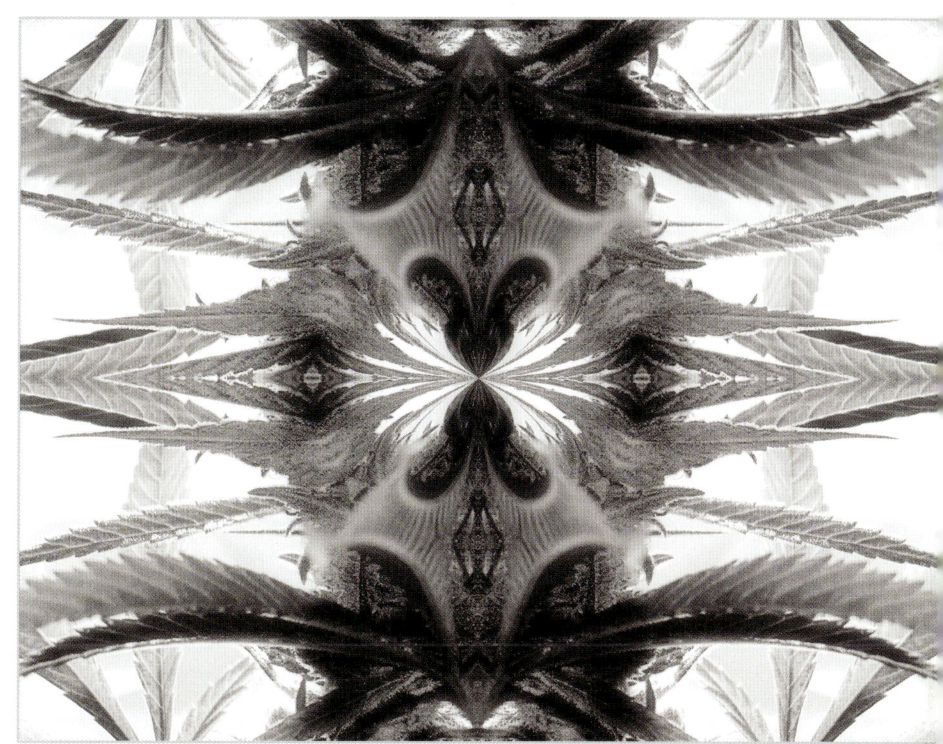

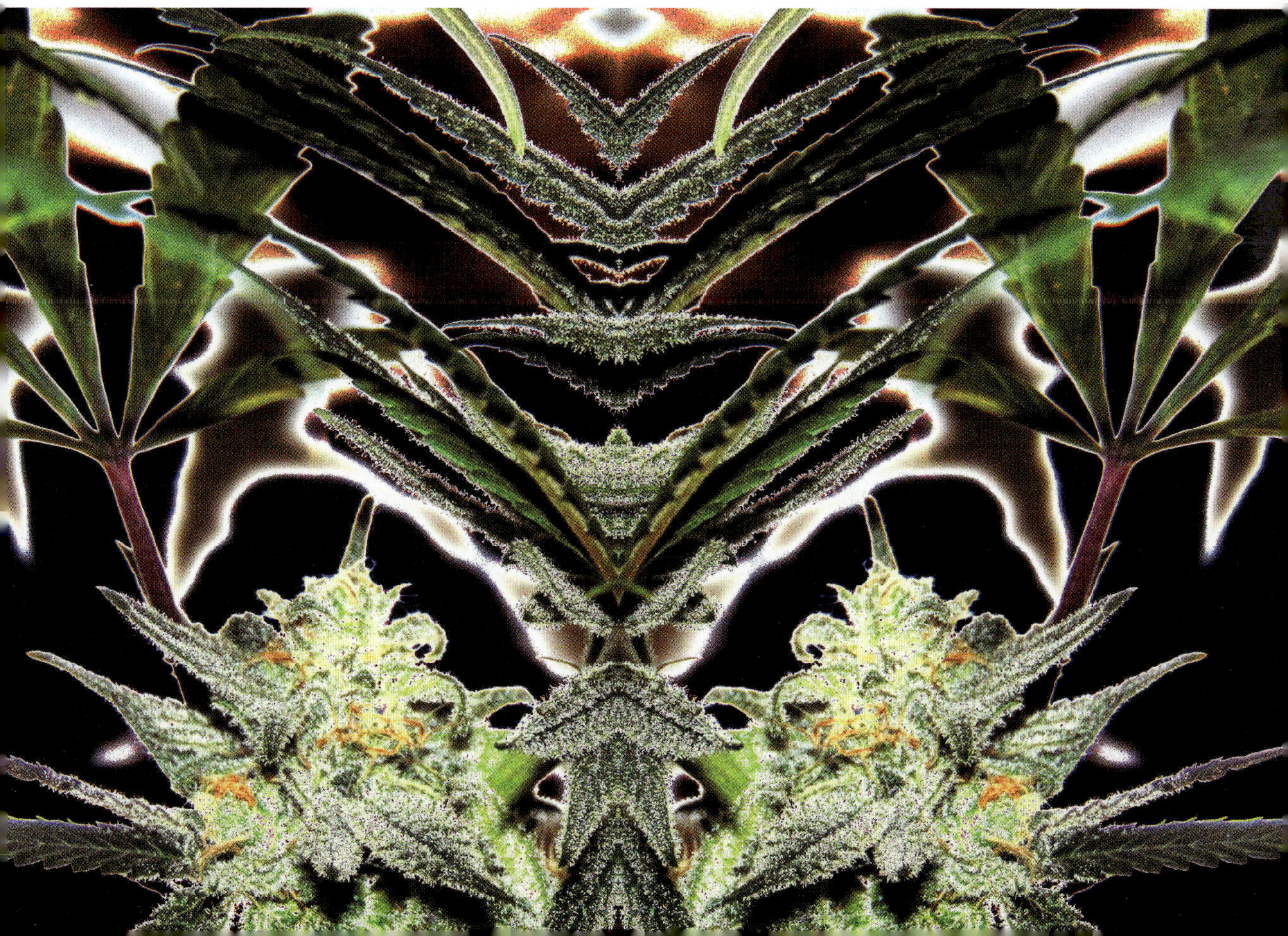

Canna-Owl

below—The canna-owl sits on his perch, looking at you looking at him. I would advise you to hold very still. If he lunges at you, he will stick to your face!

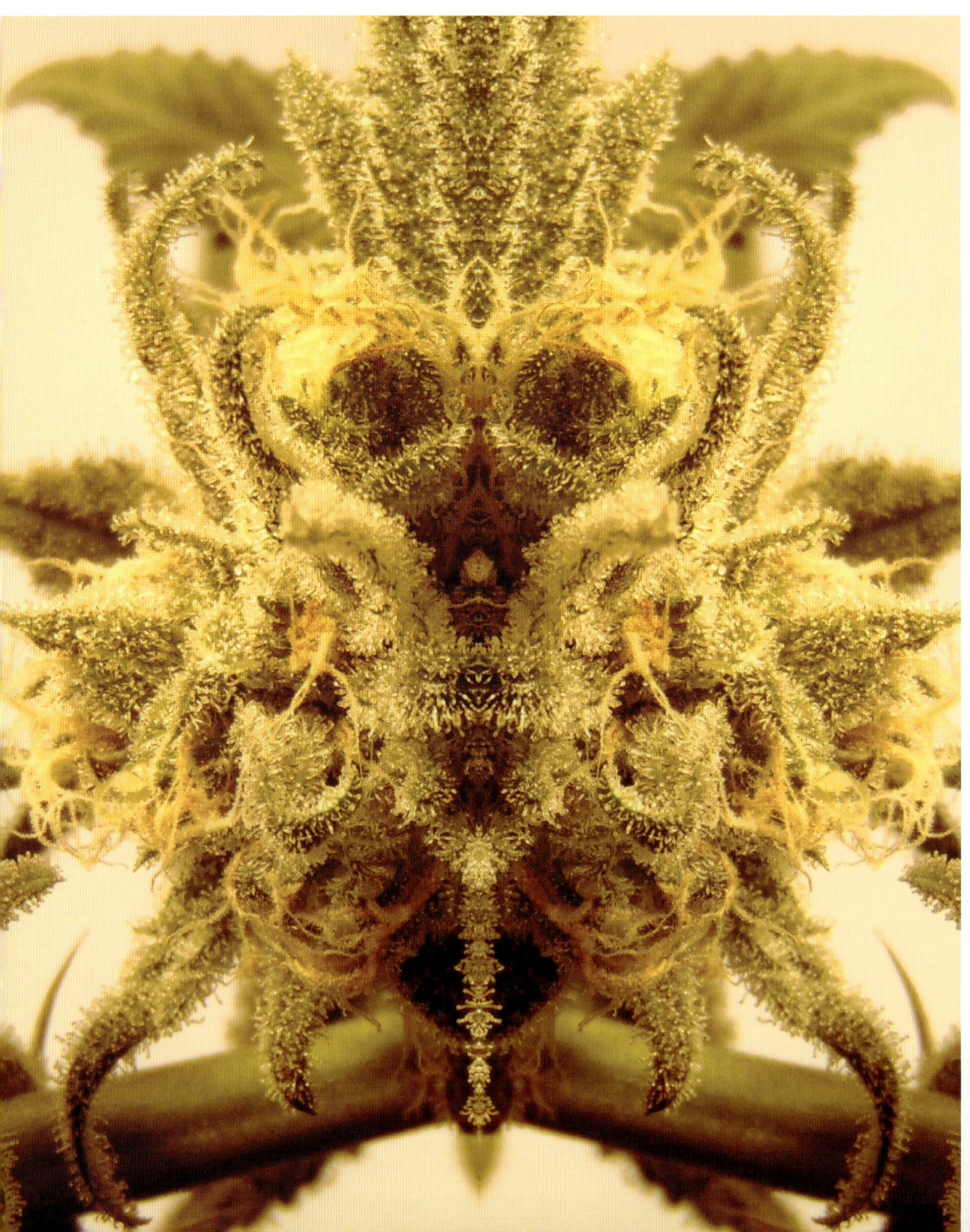

right—Remember those images that people get you to stare at, then there's a loud noise and an image pops up and scares the bejesus out of you? That's what this image, and the previous one, remind me of.

below—This is what appears below the branch the owl in the image above is sitting on. I love the way the trichomes are silhouetted against the off-white background. My wife sees dinosaurs holding up the branch for the owl. It appears they are supporting a few cool creatures that the owl caught with his sticky tongue.

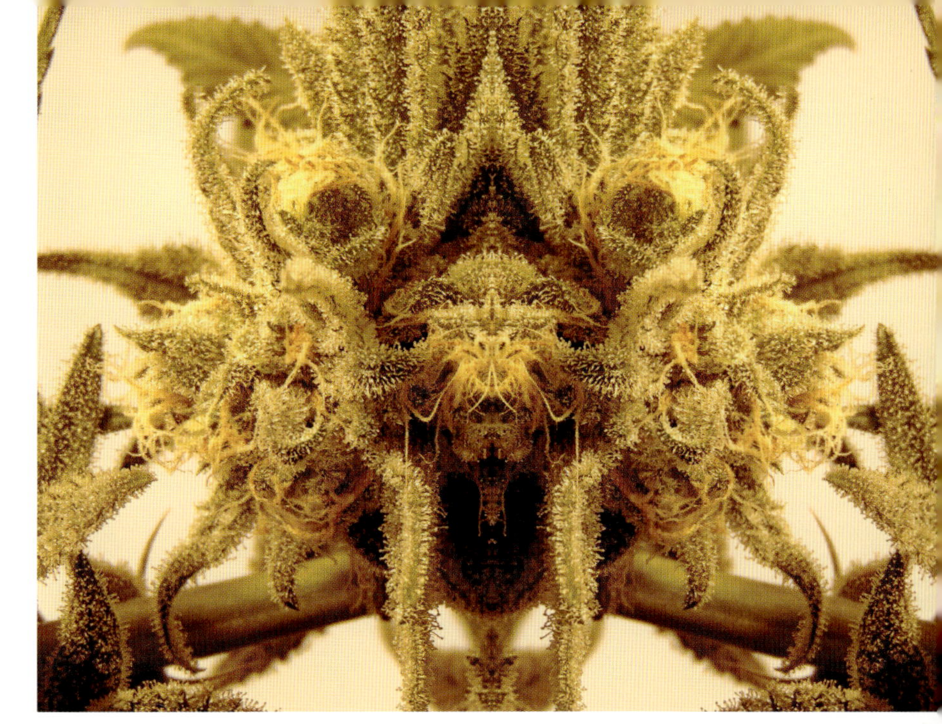

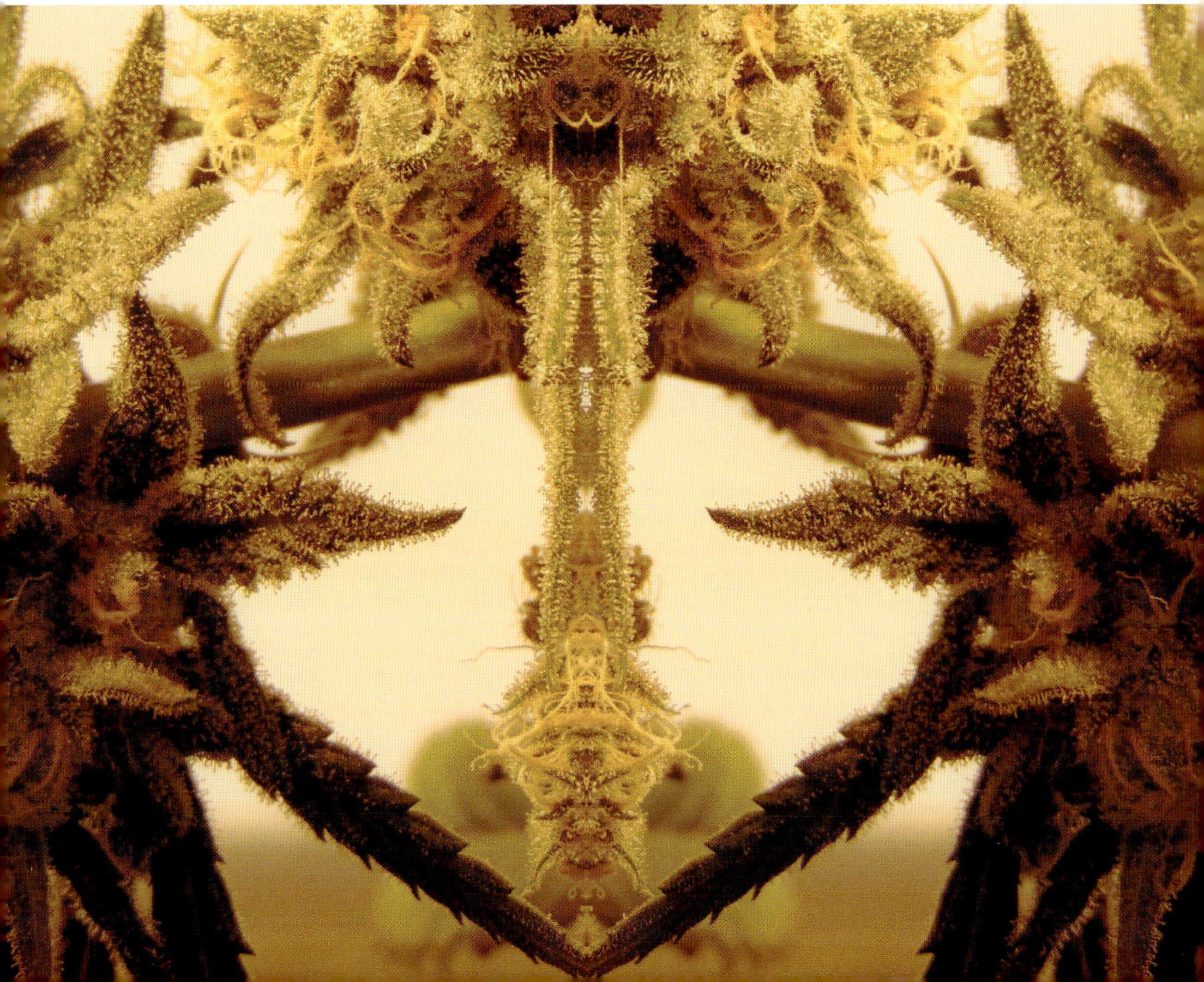

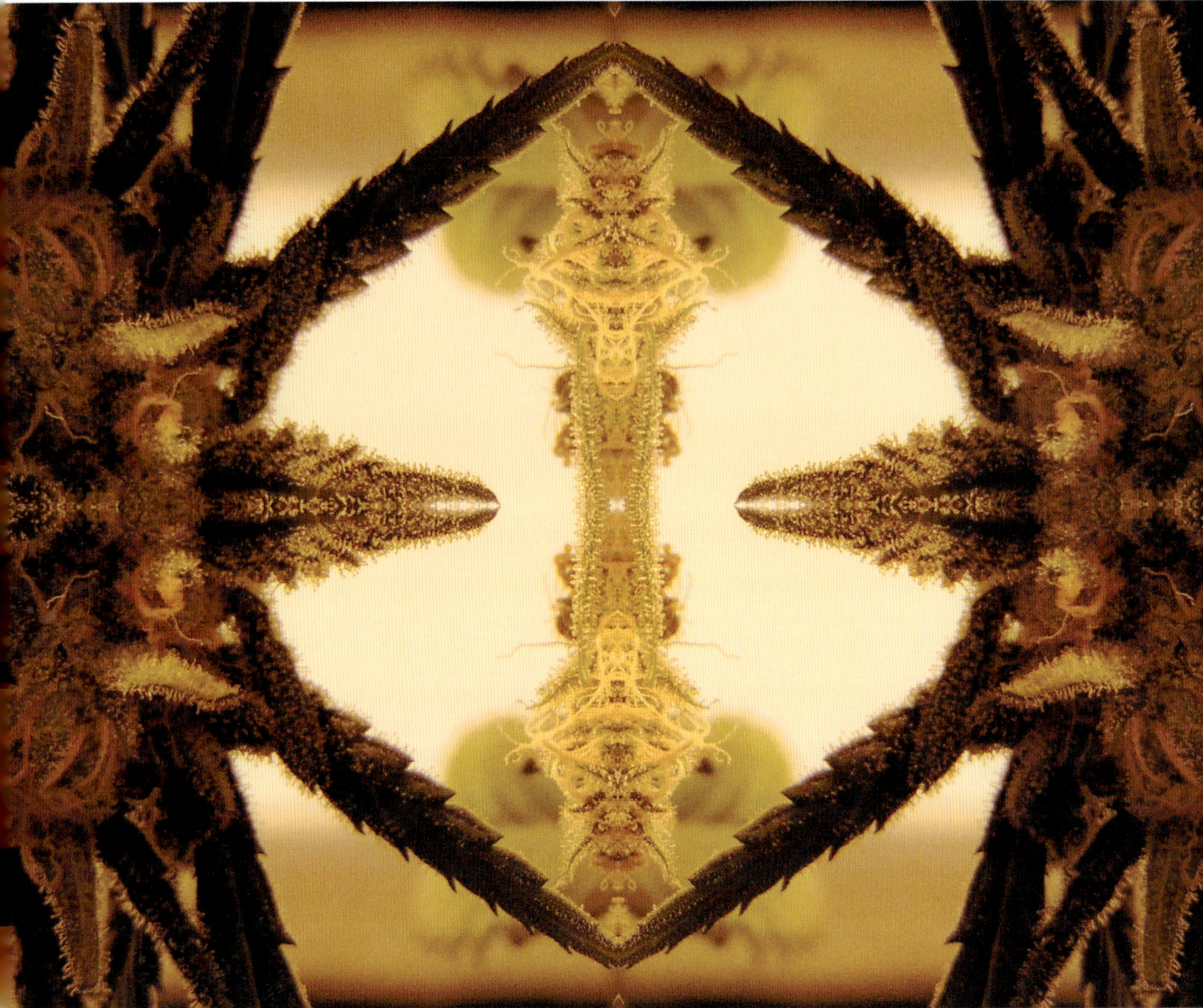

Another Vision

above—To create this image, I rotated the
previous image 90 degrees, mirrored it again,
then brought it back to a horizontal format.
We now have a top view of the dinosaur beings
stretching the creatures to show detail of the
catch on a horizontal plane. They hold together because they are so sticky.

Inspiration

right—This is the original image used to create many of the shots in this series. It's really cool to get so many image options from just one photo.

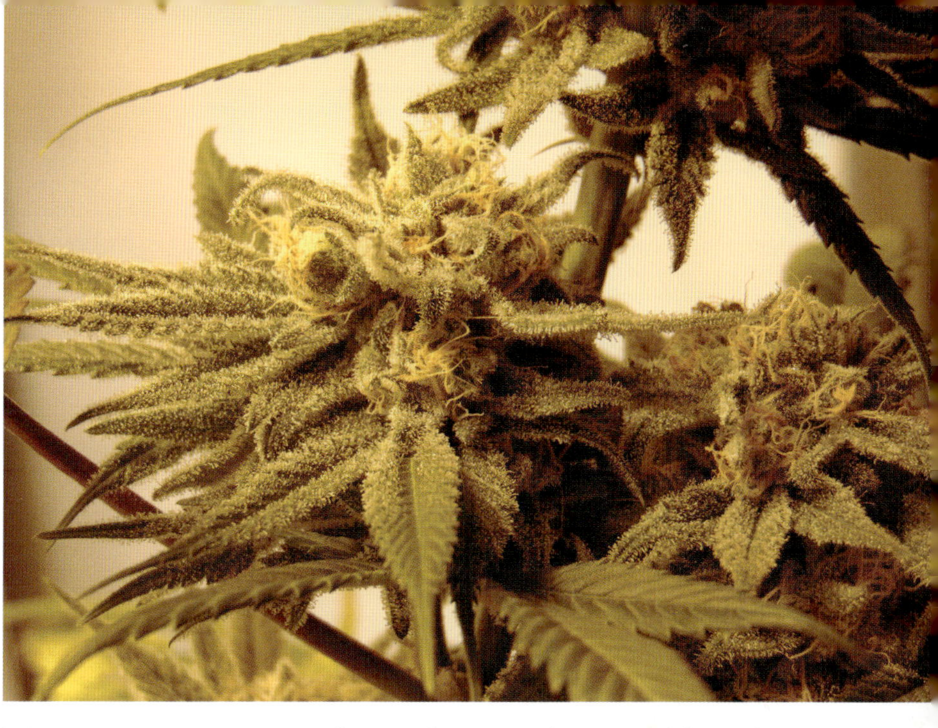

Contempt

below—The head in the center is that of a mad canna-being. He's angry that his family has been shunned since prohibition against them was established. They were bullied, condemned, and killed in an effort to eradicate them from the face of the earth. Innocent people were beaten and separated from their families to be put in jails and prisons. He is growing stronger every day, calling attention to his family's importance.

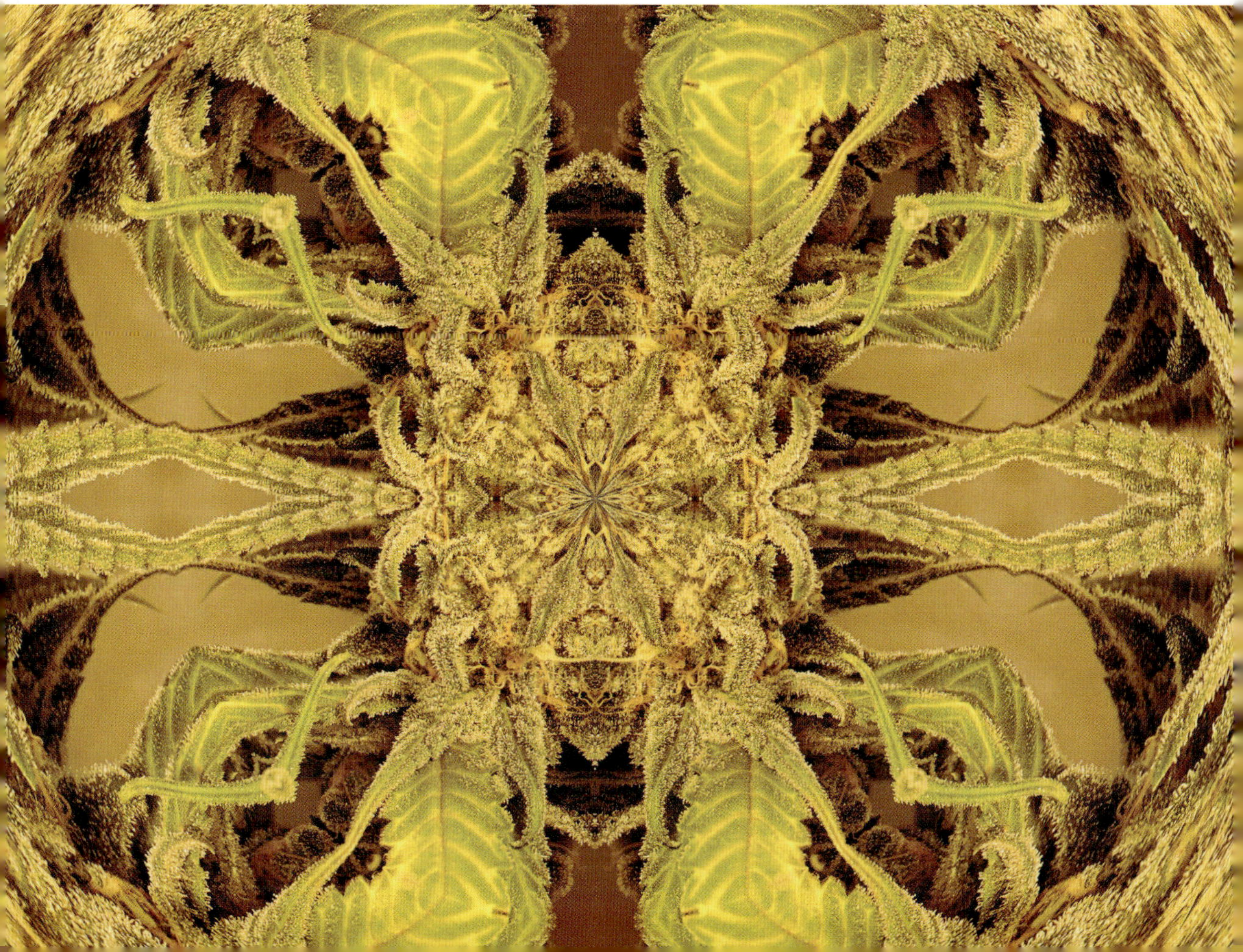

Smile!

top—As a whole and down the center, this image has many cool aspects to make you smile.

Make Your Own

bottom—Come up with your own caption for this one. What do you see?

Bridge

following page—Many people see this as a giant spider looking down on a very sticky bridge. I can see why. I also see two elephants, plus some trumpeter elephants starting to cross the bridge. I hope it can take the weight!

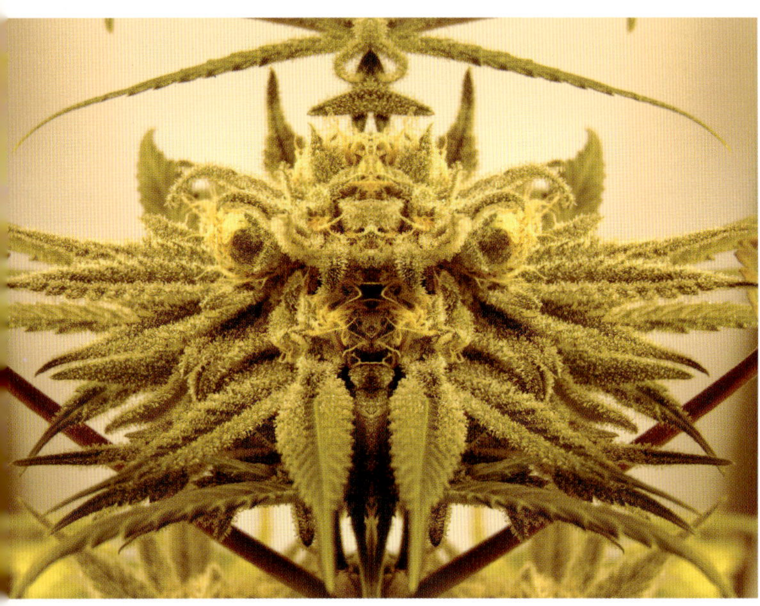

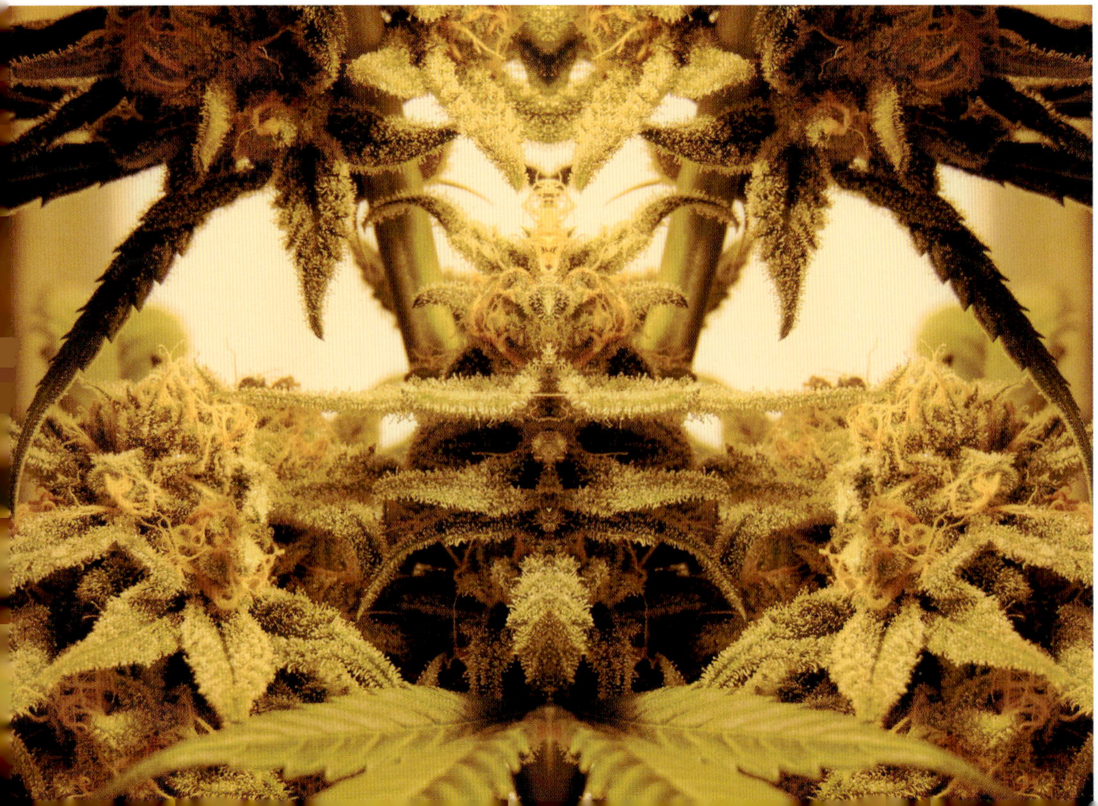

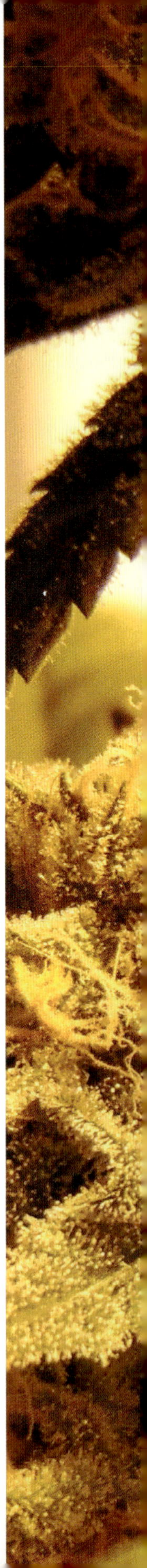

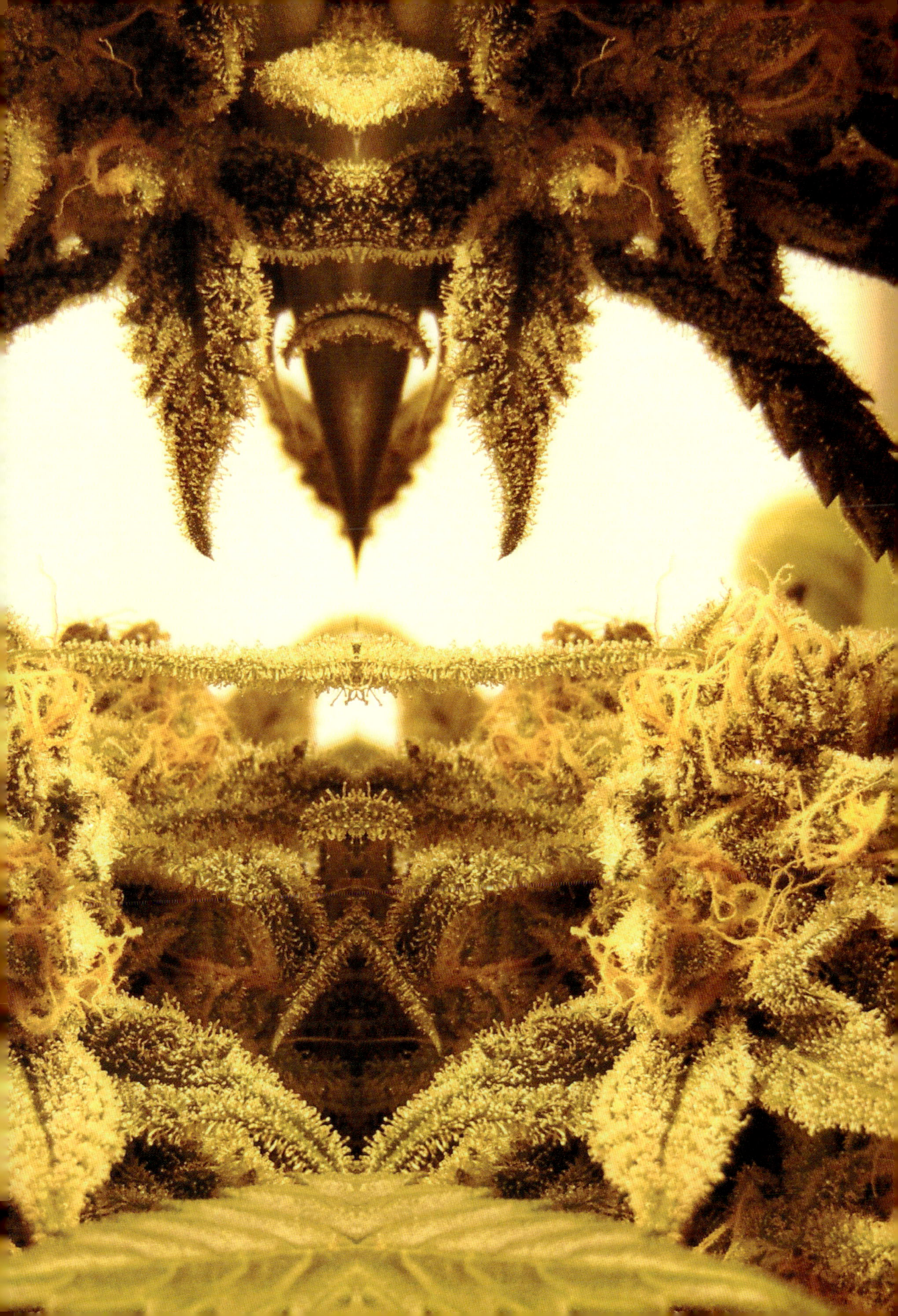

Experimentation

below and following page—The images on this page spread were made from the same original image. Playing with images in postproduction can be a lot of fun. I've discovered many creative options just by clicking around in my editing program, experimenting, and finding my way. The image below is a six-petal kaleidoscope.

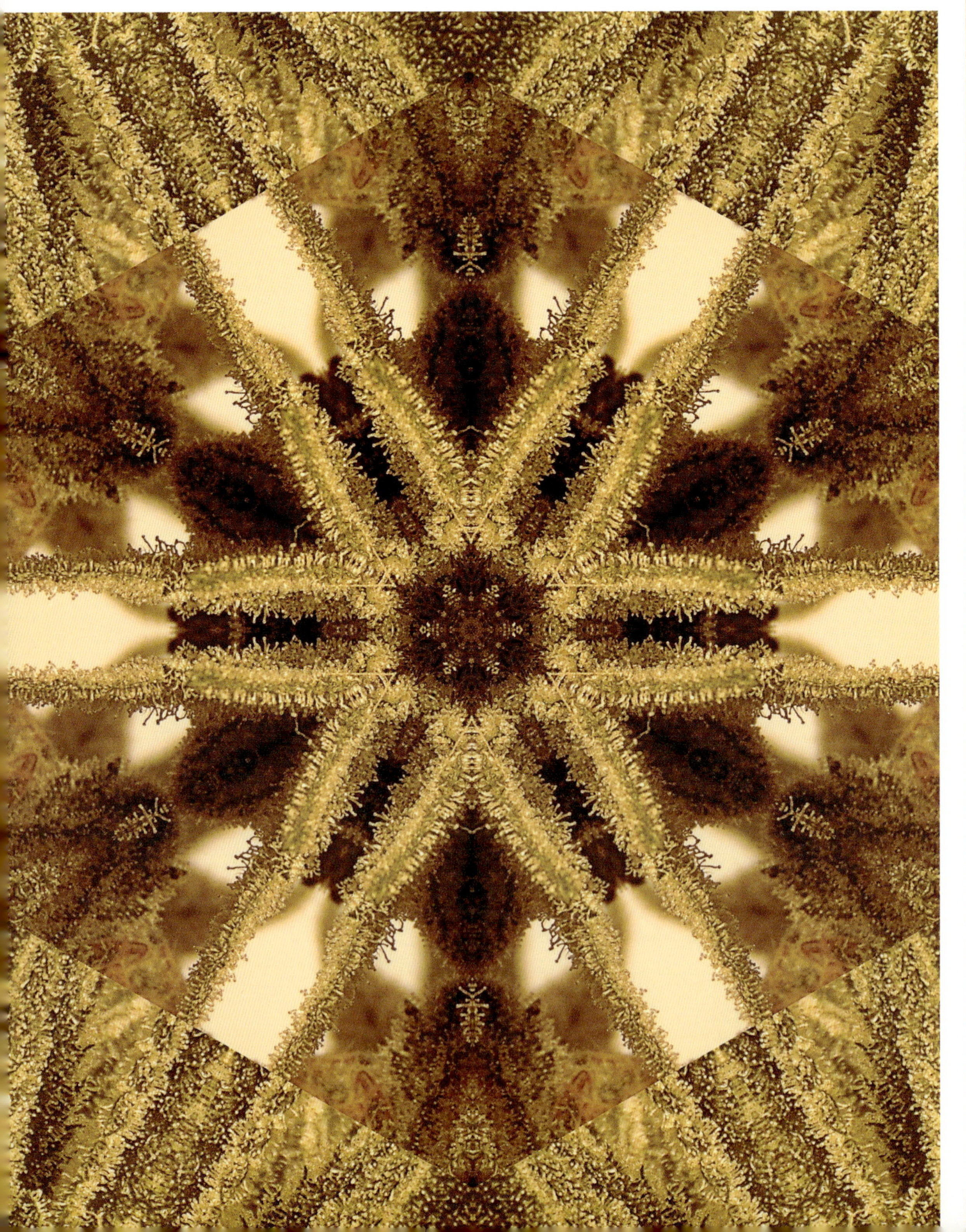

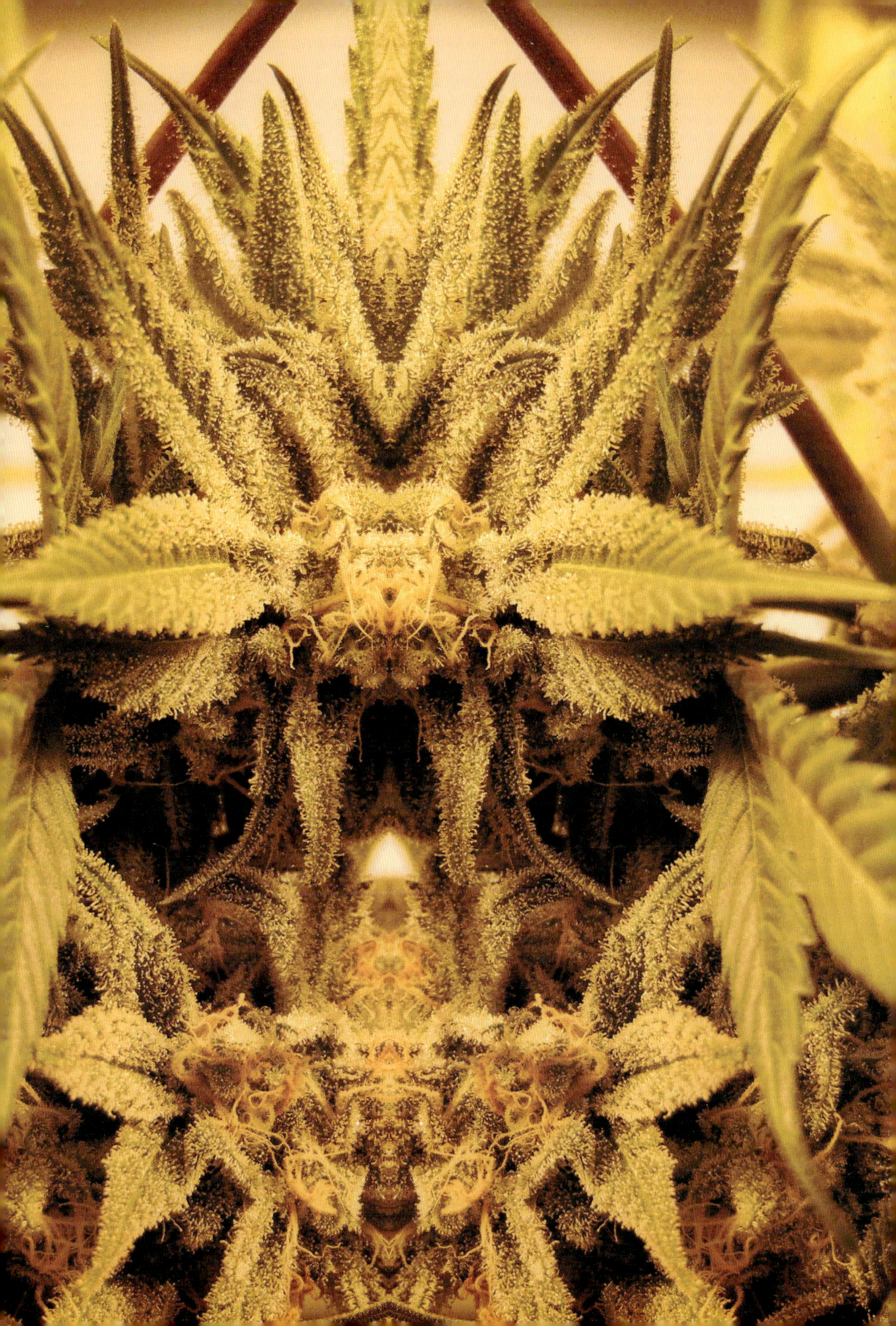

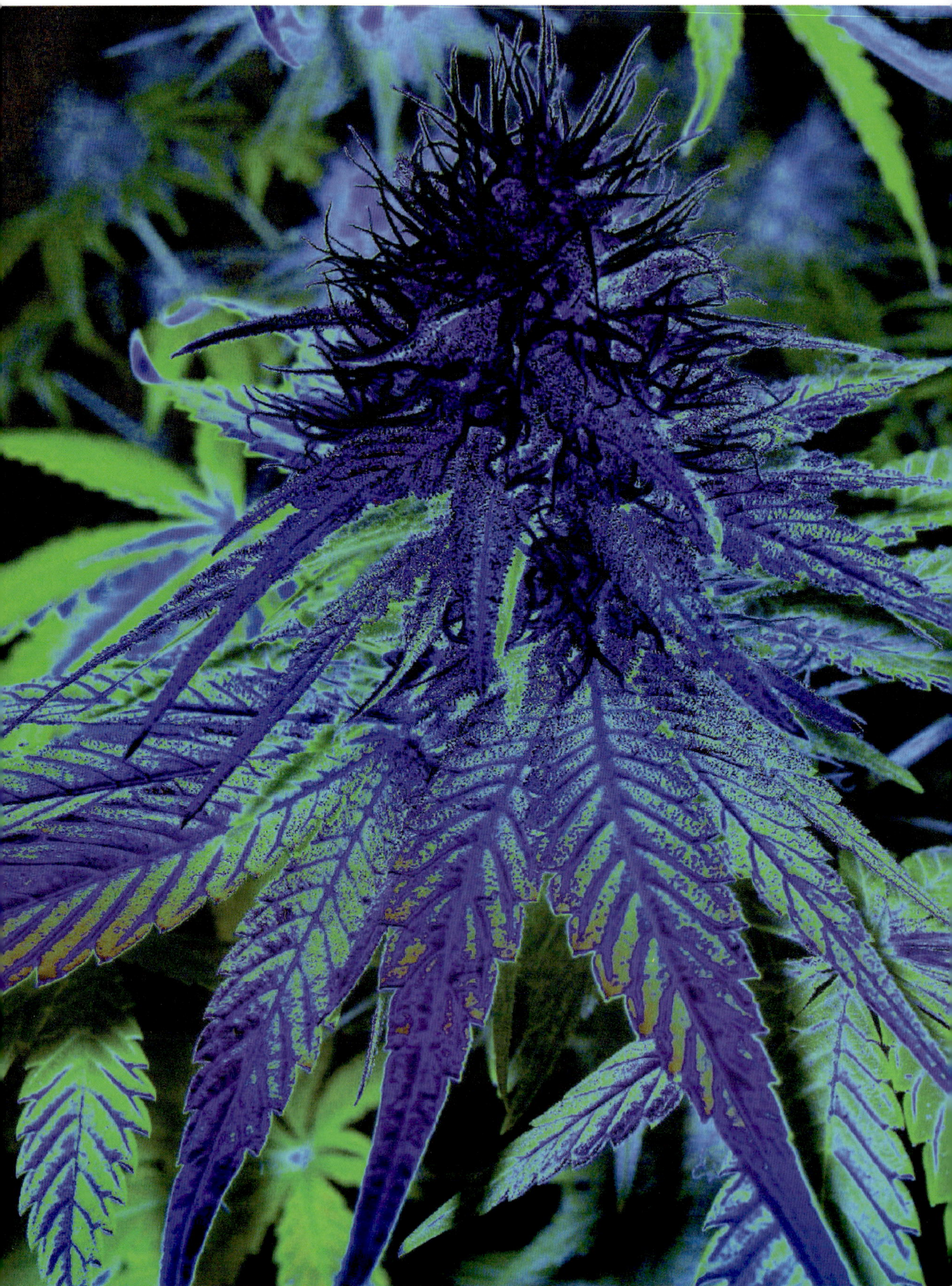

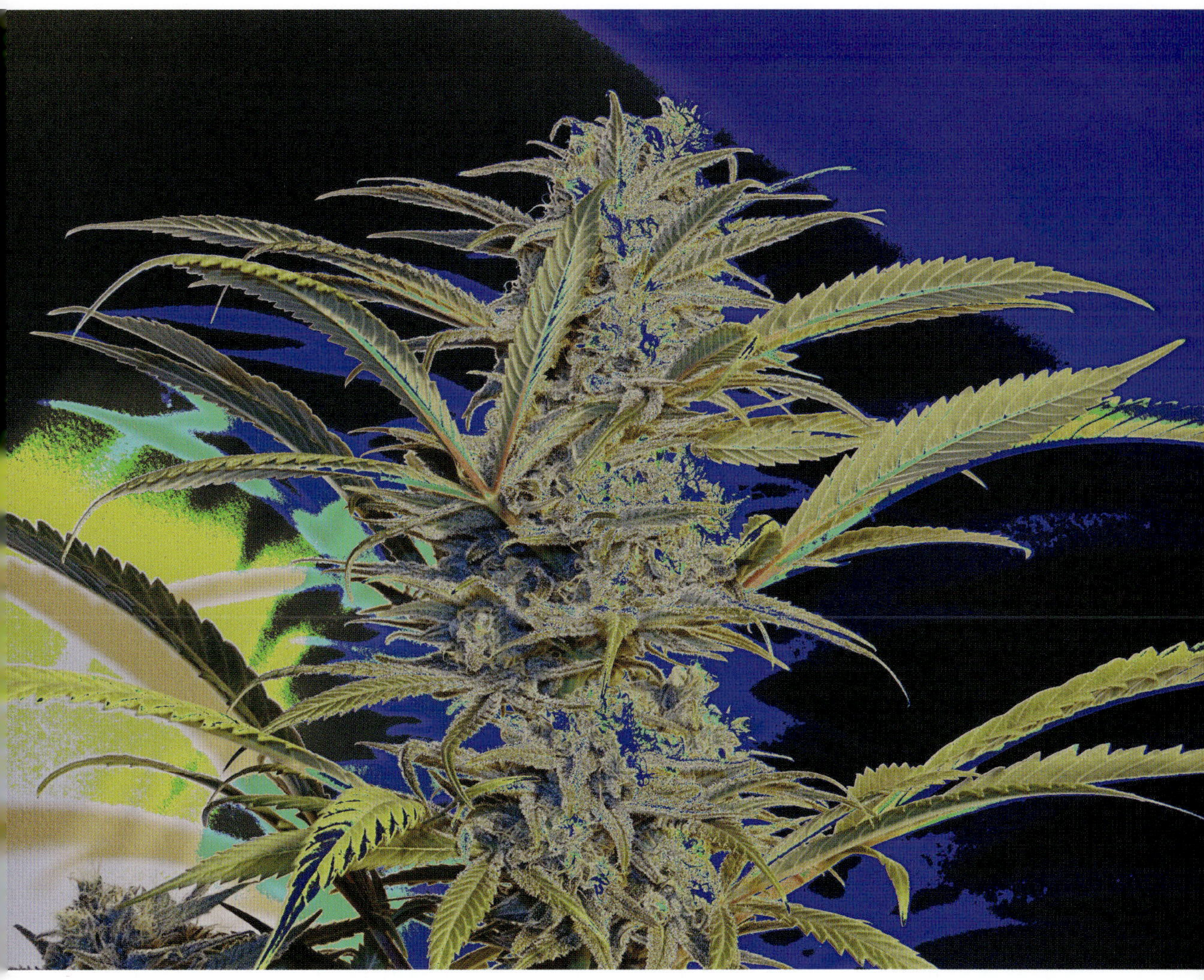

A Punch of Color

previous page—Here's a color-altered photograph of a nice Blue Dream bud, reduced to blue, black, and green. The buds in the background mimic the one in the foreground.

Aztec

above—Some people think this photograph has an Aztec look to it. The colors filled in an odd way, but I think it made for a unique image.

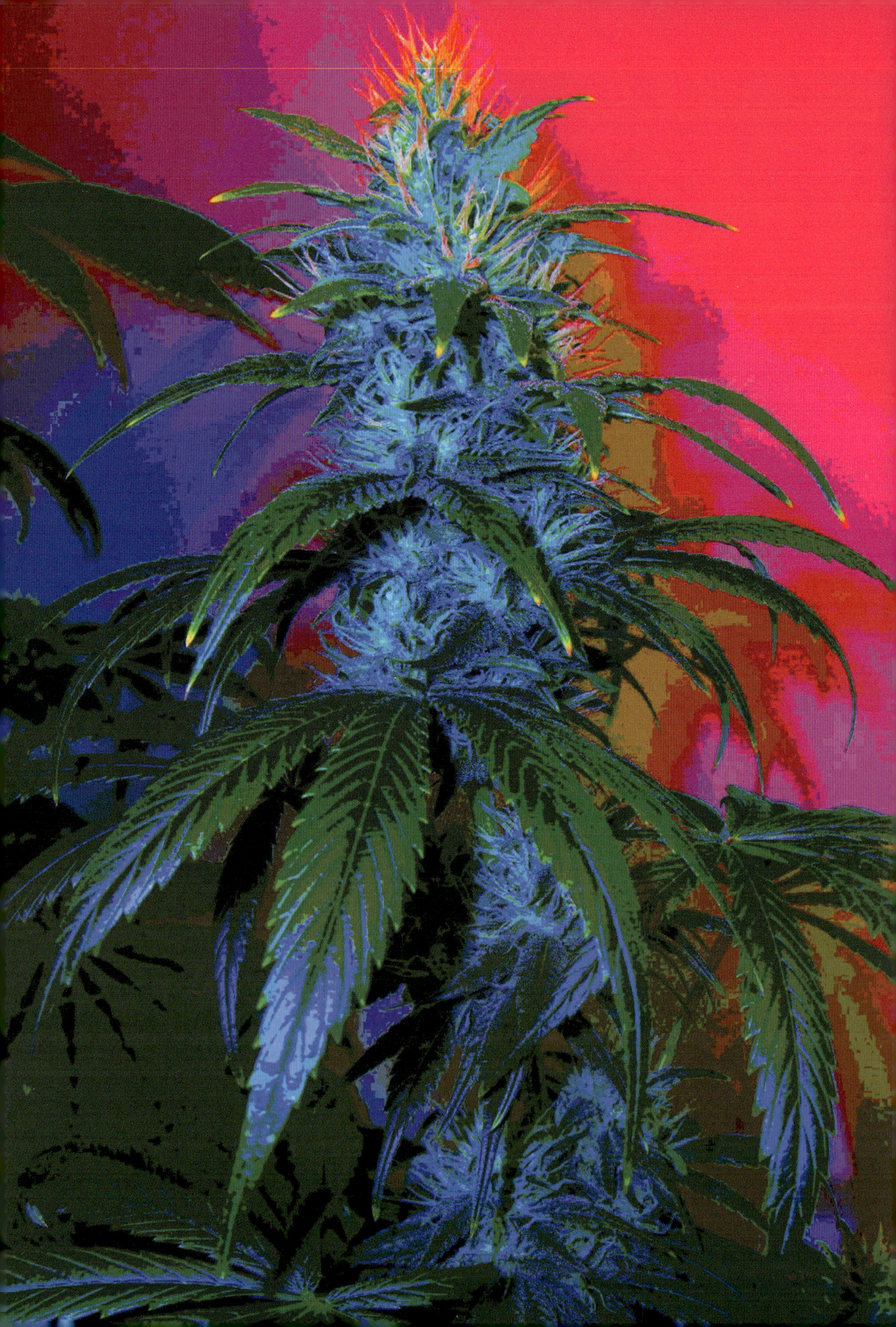

Altered Reality

Here are a few more color-altered images.

previous page—This is a Blue Dream cola. She's been flowering for about three-and-a-half weeks at this point.

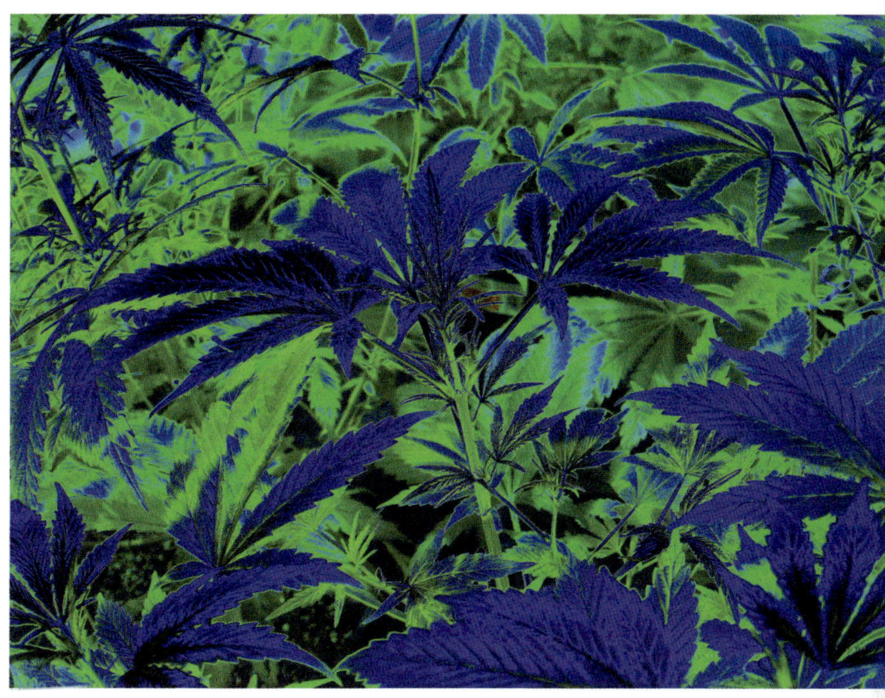

above right—Indica from seed. You can tell plants are from seed when there are consistently two nodes opposite each other. This changes at the tops after a couple weeks of flowering when they start to alternate.

below—The density of the trichomes is reflected by the saturated, dense blue in this shot. I think the contrast between the green and blue is striking.

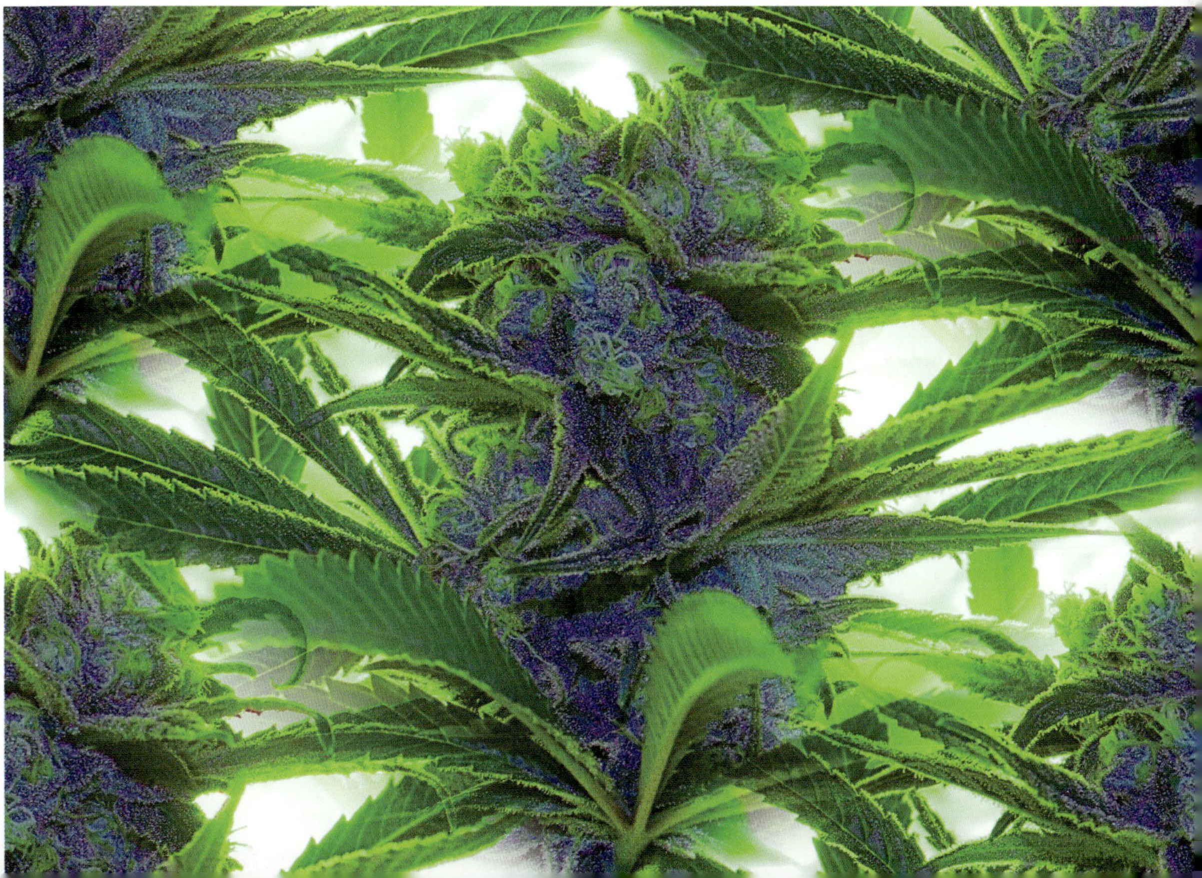

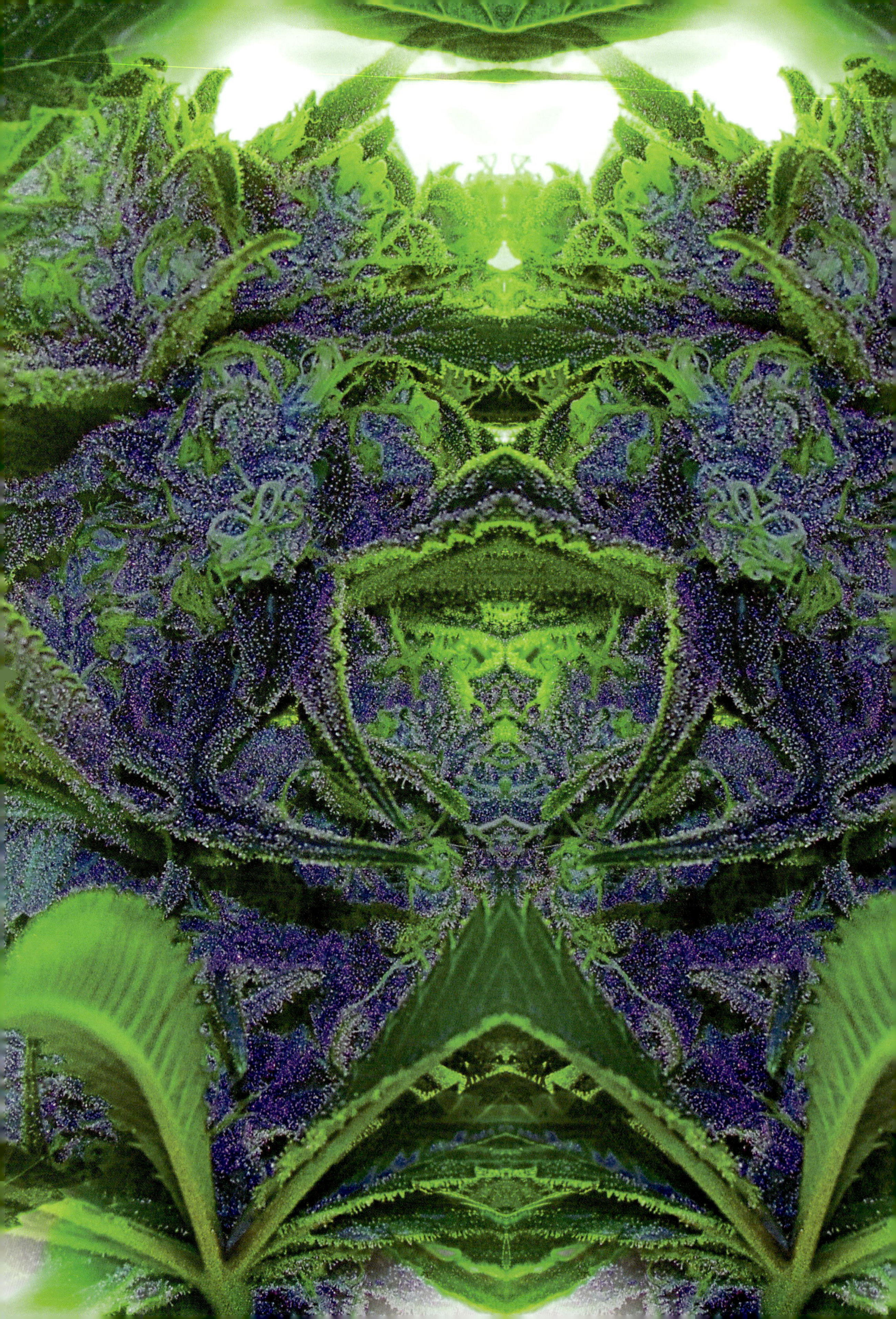

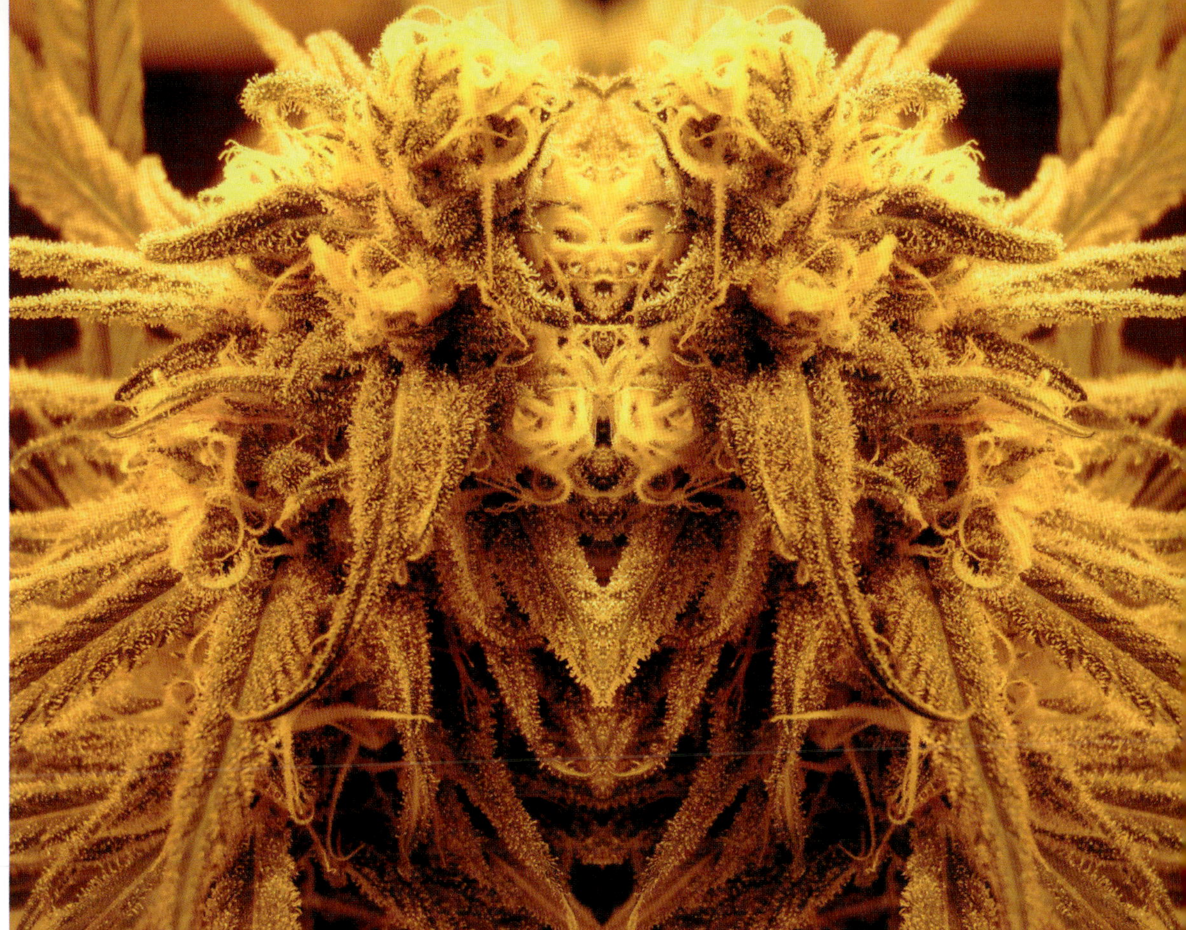

A New View

previous page—Mirroring the previous image revealed many long-armed, long-legged creatures hiding in the center. I especially like the little dude at the top with the two V-shaped hair follicles.

A Sight to Behold

above—The glands on this Blue Dream plant are amazing. Even the dude at the top has a shocked look on his face. Depending on what I want out of a particular shot, I like to photograph plants when they're about half to three-quarters mature.

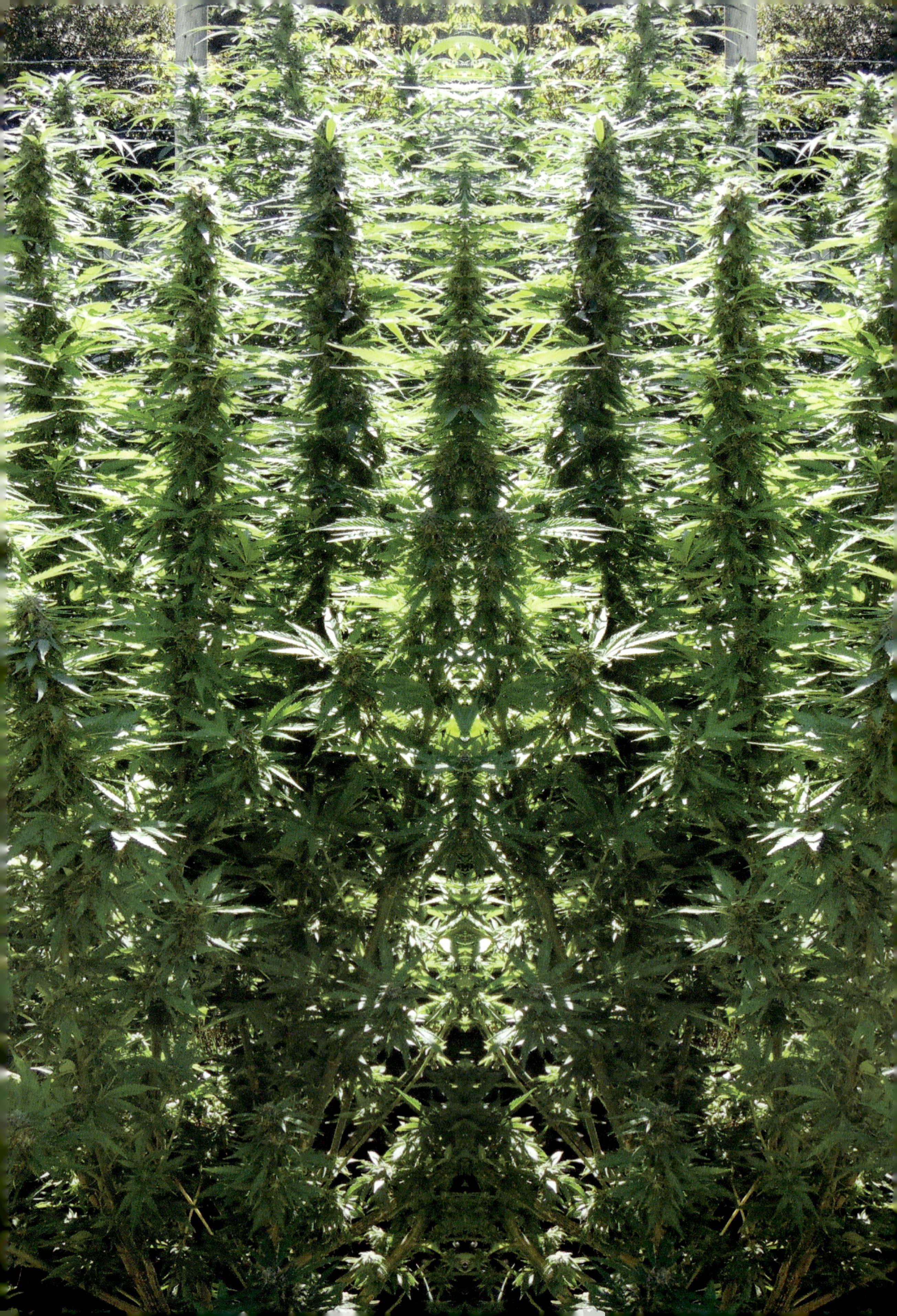

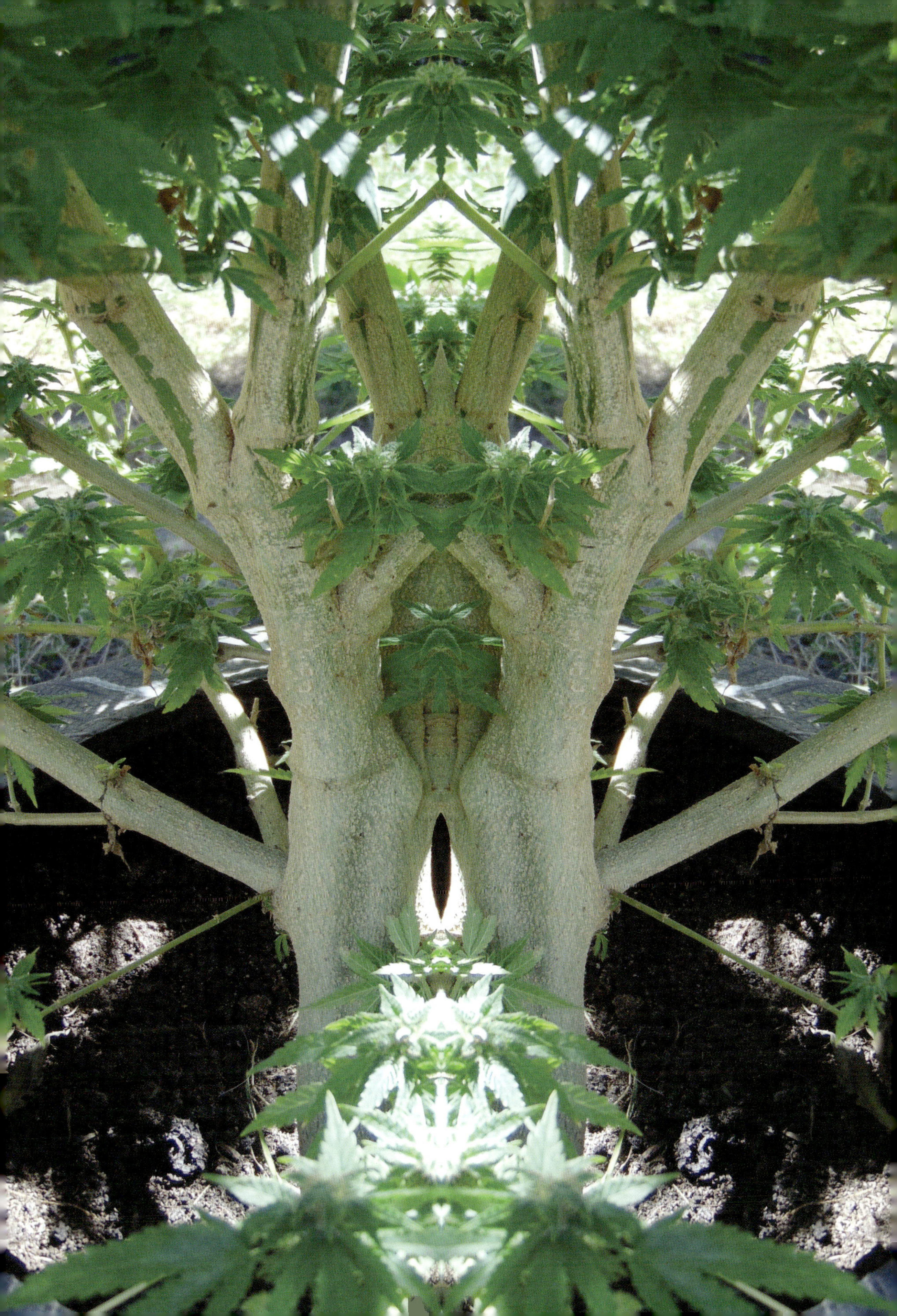

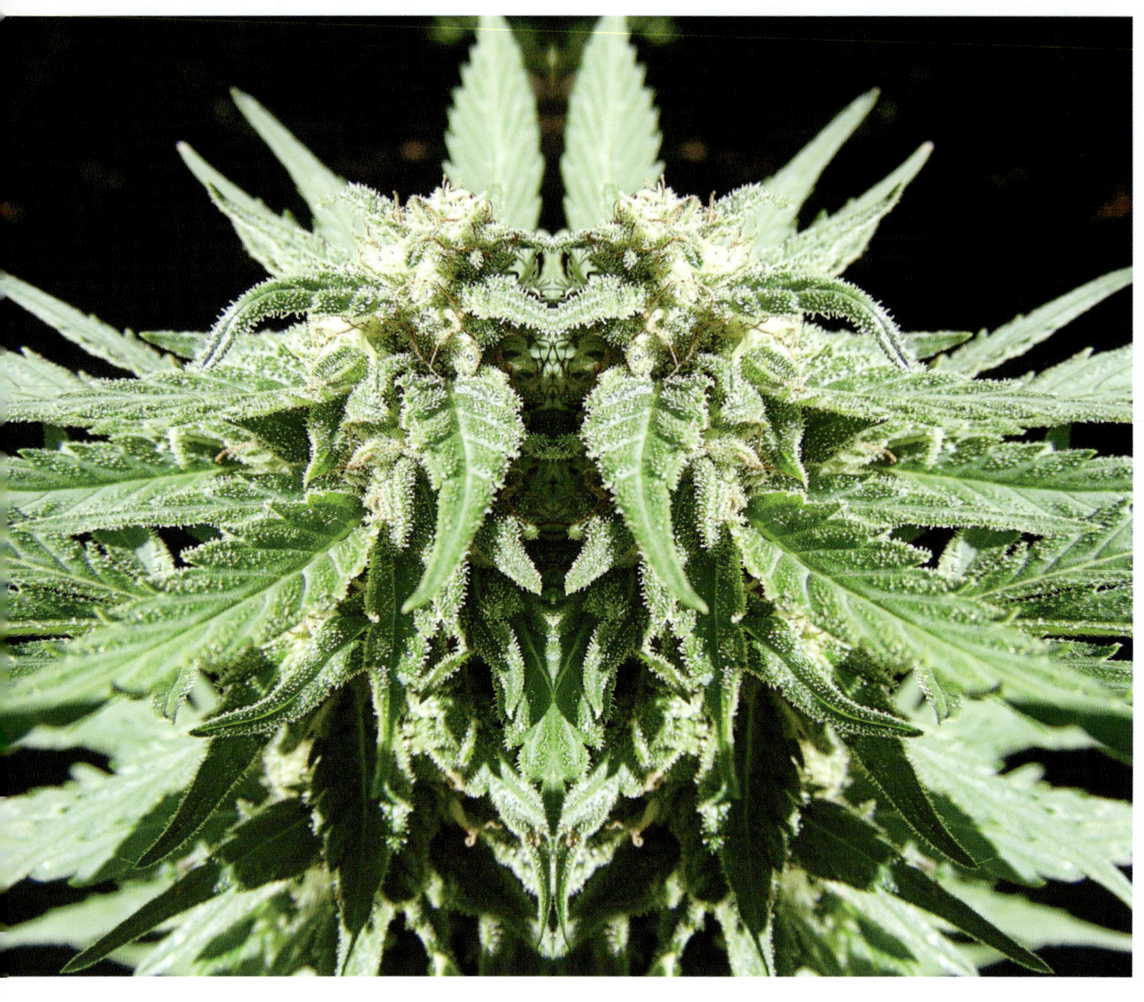

Lovely Lady

following page—If you have a good imagination, pareidolia should be starting to creep in. Your ability to recognize faces, shapes, and beings is rising as a natural response to the stimuli entering your brain. Kick back and set it free.

At the dead center of the image, you can see a ballerina's pointed feet. As you look upward, you'll find a blue spot; it's the bottom of her dress, poofed out at the knees. Above her hips, you can see her arms stretched out and angled downward. There's a smile on her face. Her headress turns into another being's mouth.

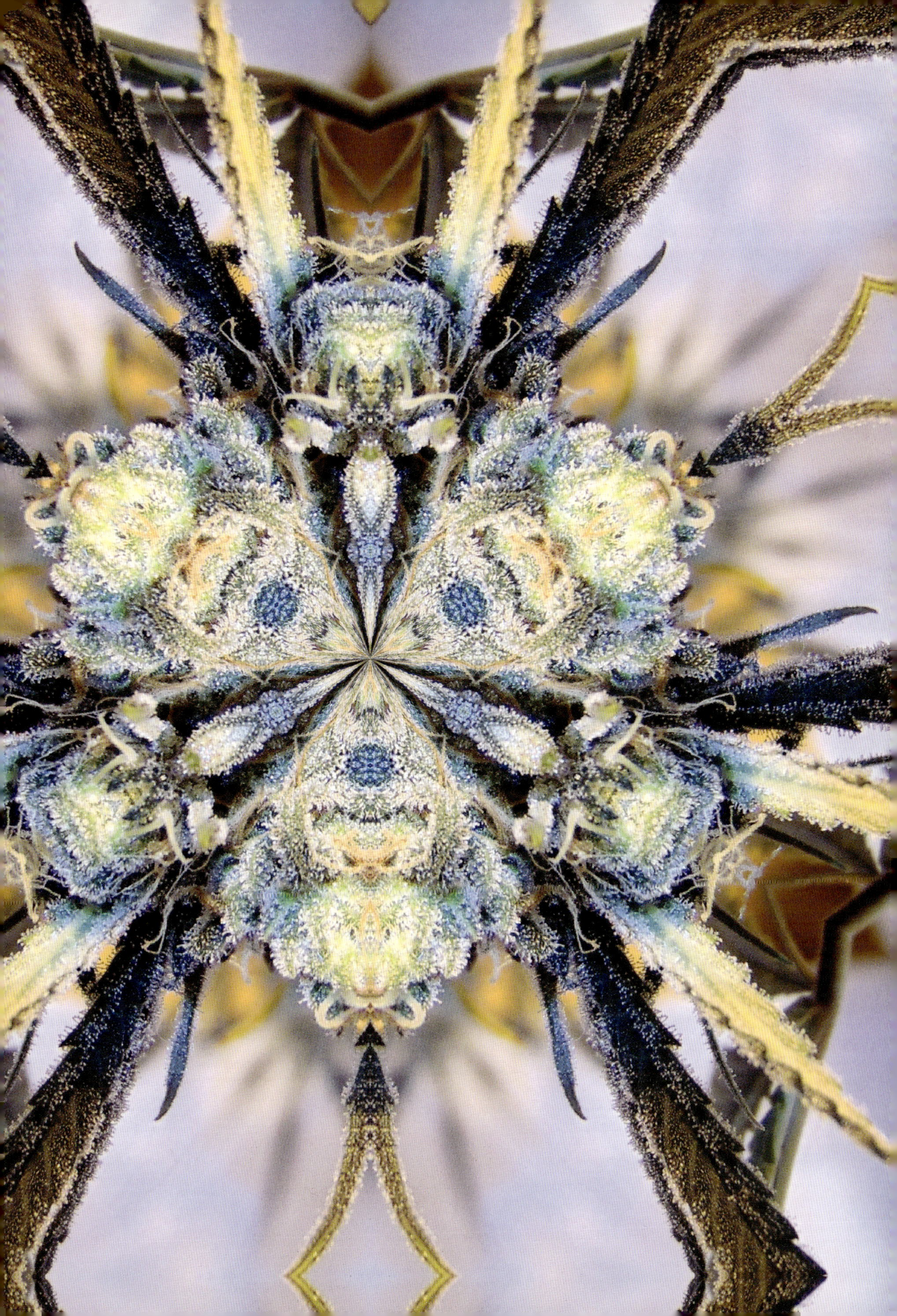

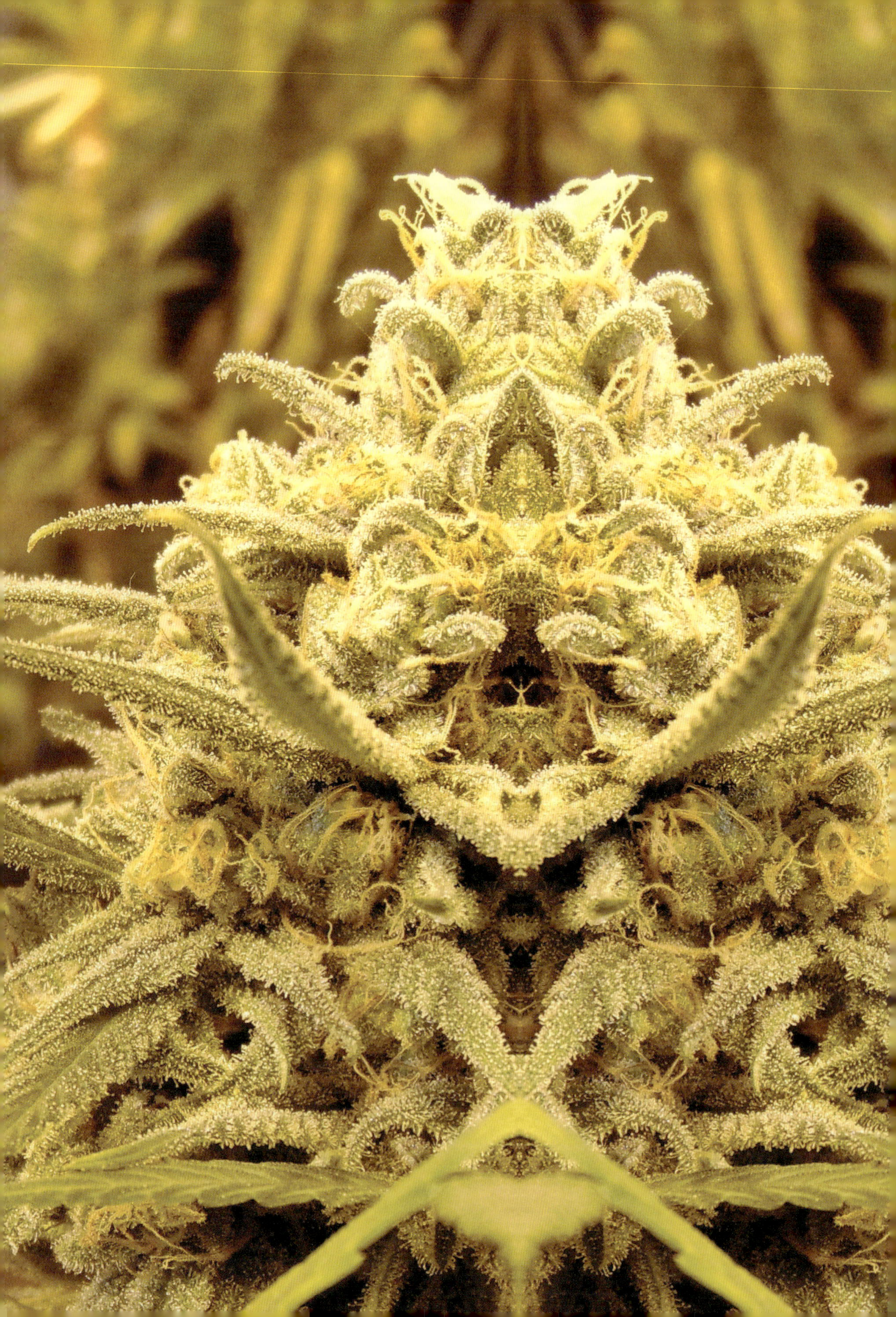

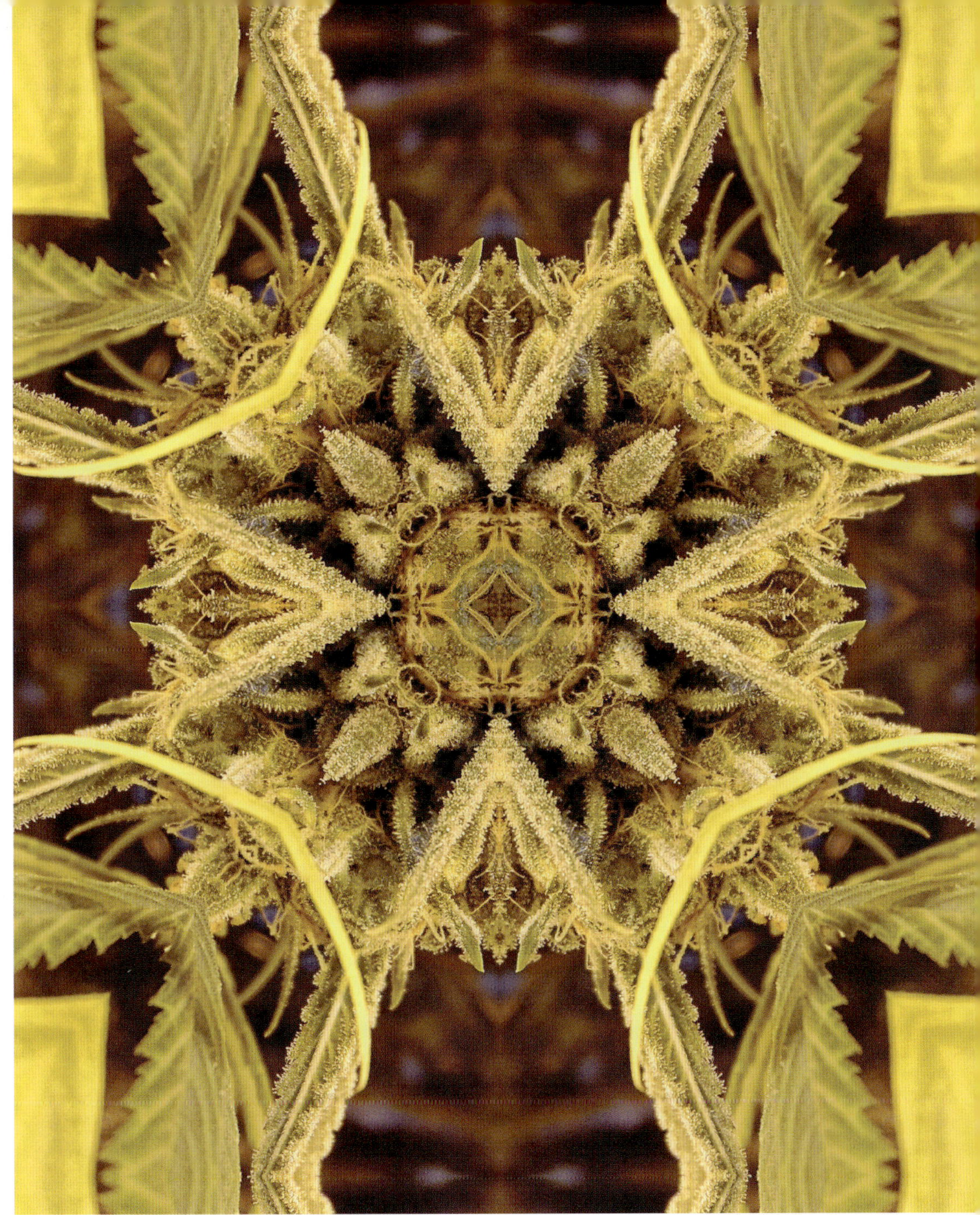

Cathedral

above—When I look at this image, I imagine I am looking up through a clear ceiling. I can see four round pillars rising into the air, reaching not to a cathedral ceiling, but to a platform below that. The bottom is intricately painted to draw your attention to the detail in the center.

From a Distance

below—As I mentioned earlier, many of these photographs should be viewed from a distance. This is one of those images. If you can, look at this one from a distance of about five feet.

When you do, you'll notice that some of the details become lost in the background, and new forms take shape.

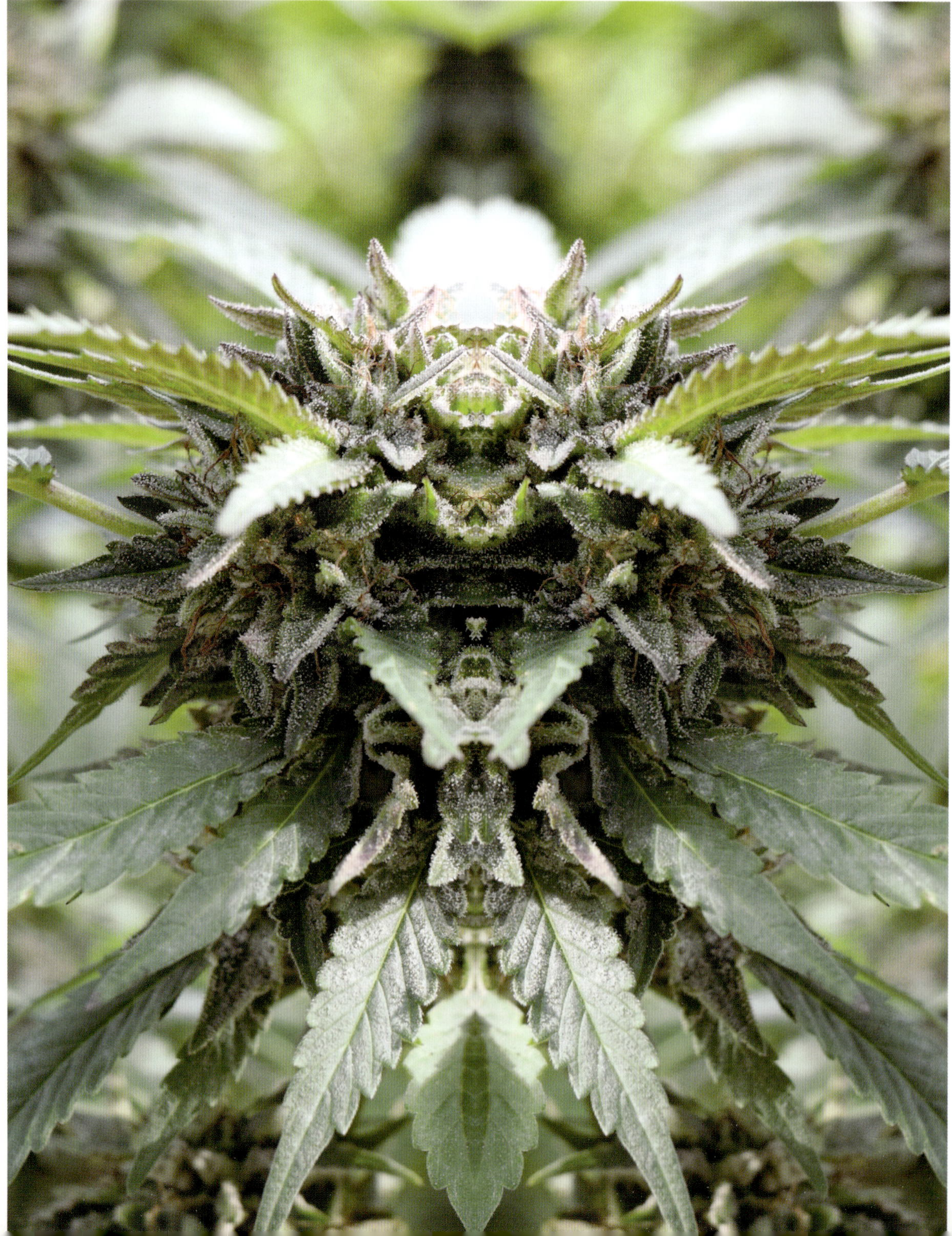

The Original

top—This is the original image that I used for the next three photographs. As you can see, each one is wonderfully different from the last.

Lionlike

bottom—Mirroring the previous image surprised me. The face in the middle has been interpreted in many different ways, but I see it as a lion. There are other faces that peek out, too. I get a laugh from the one at the top, because it reminds me of Marvin the Martian from the Bugs Bunny cartoons.

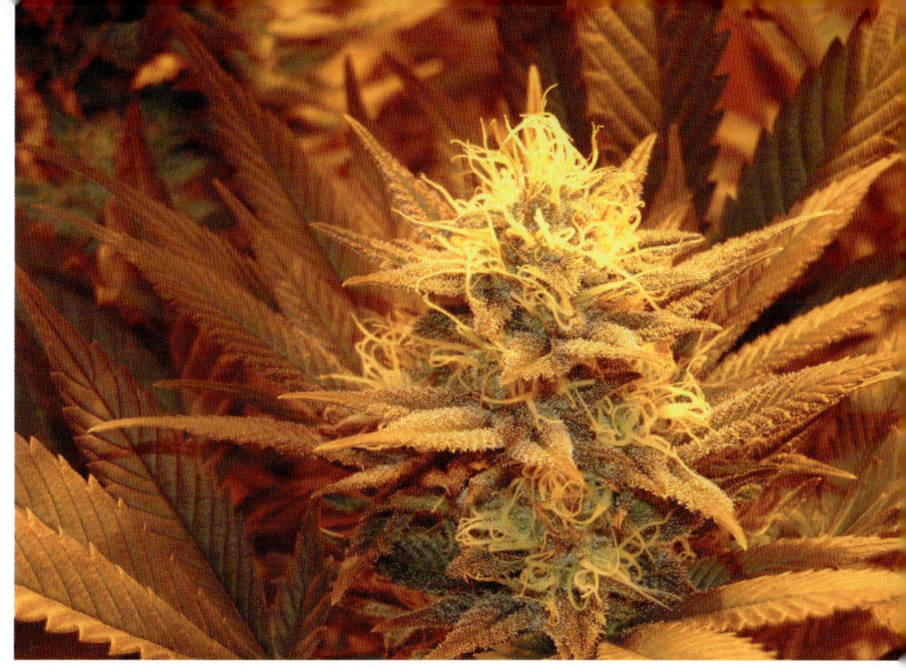

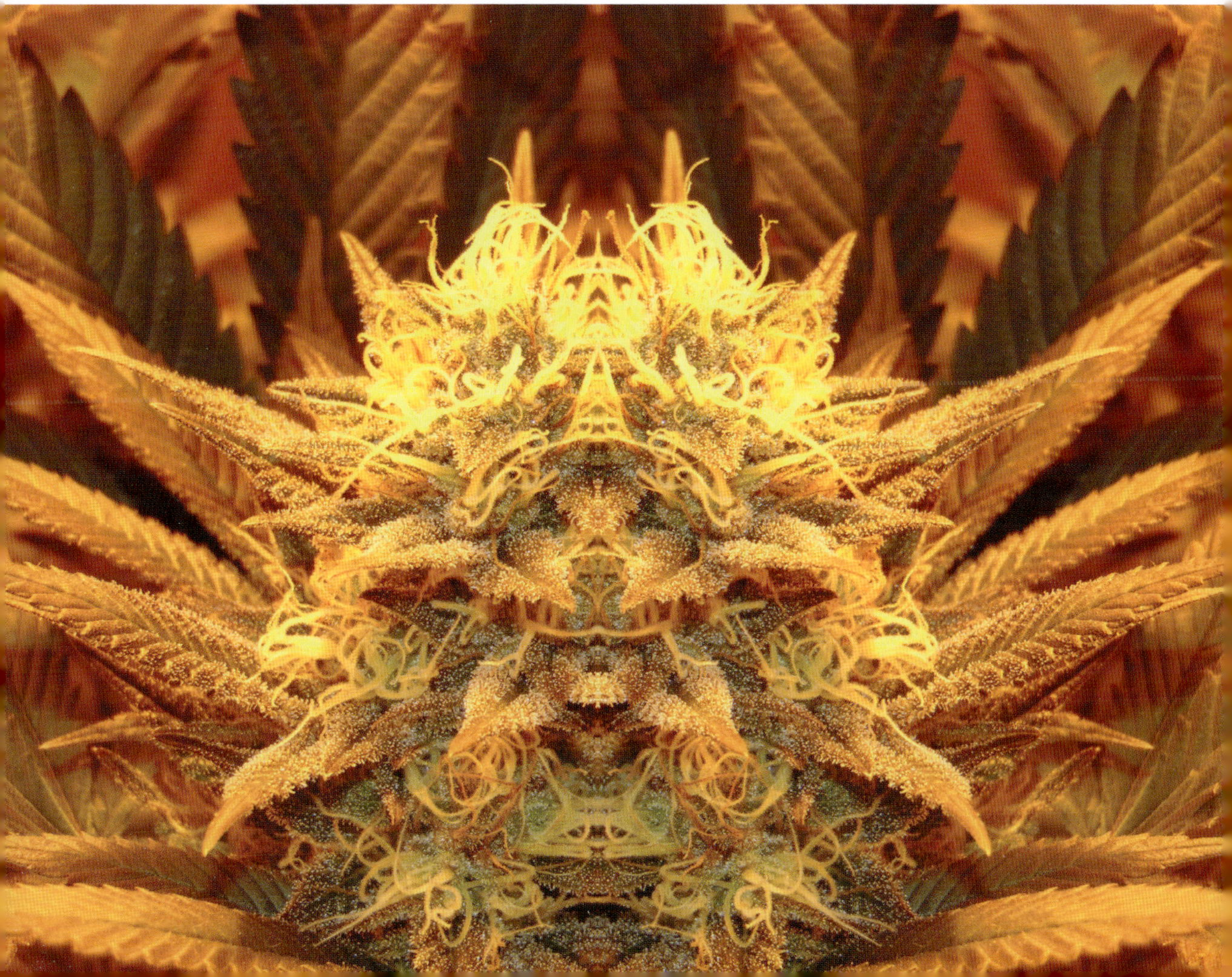

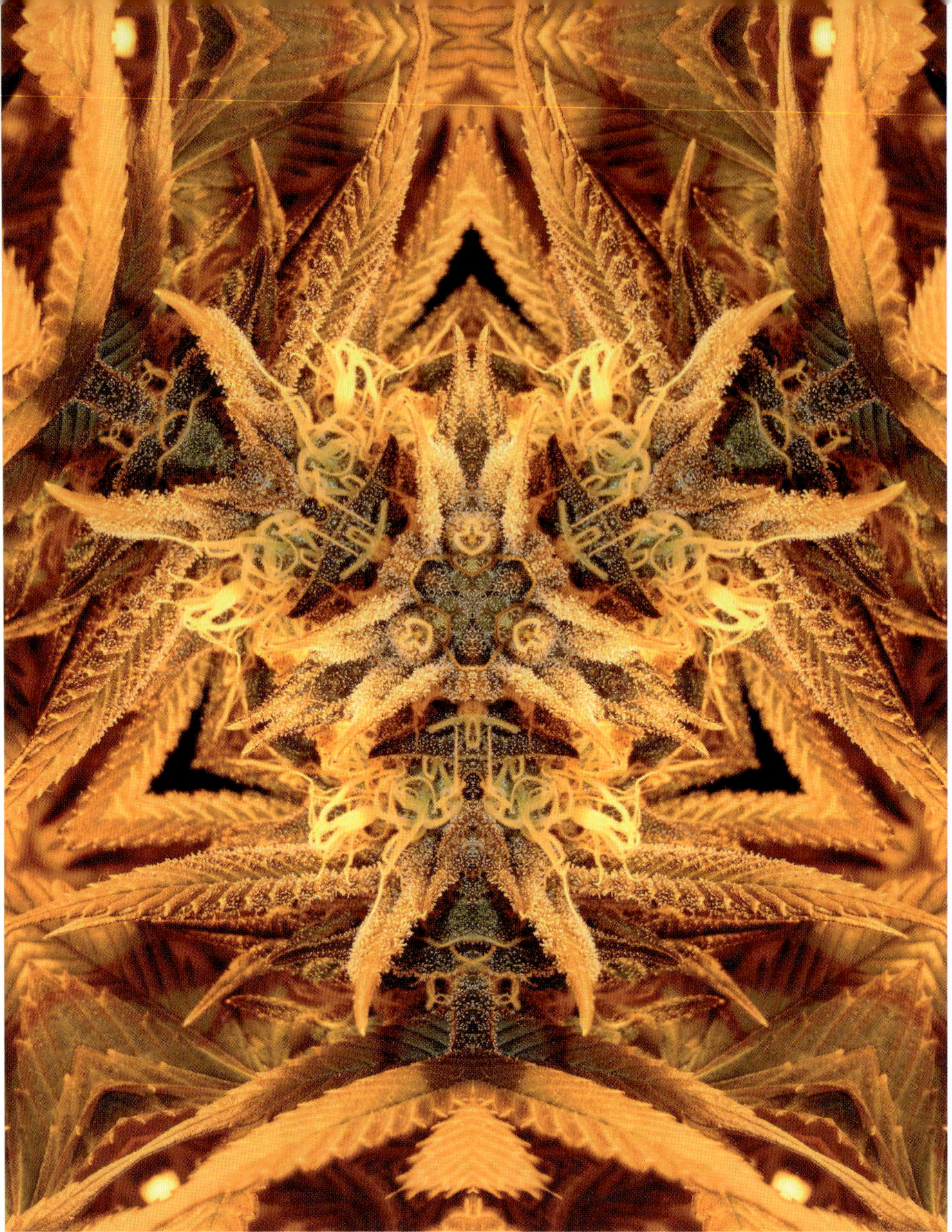

Smiling Lady

above—Three-petal kaleidoscope. Notice the smiling lady's face just above center of the image.

A Happy Gathering

following page—Six-petal kaleidoscope. There are six ladies sitting around a table in this rendition of the image. It's not just ladies that I see; I also see a group of jokers sitting around a table with their tongues sticking out. They are massaging the ladies' shoulders. I also see some broad-winged bird beings above their heads! I love the violet and green tones in the middle.

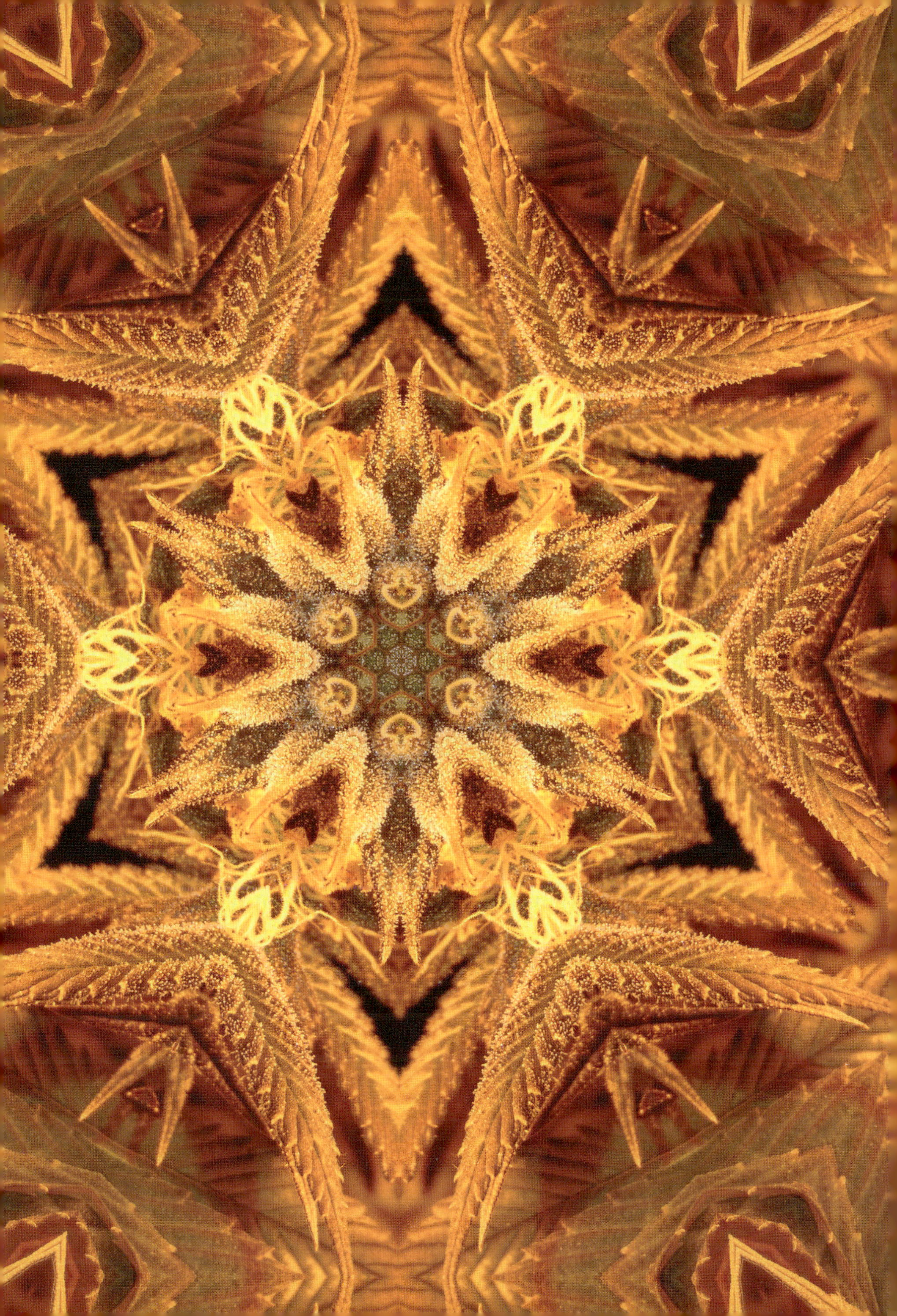

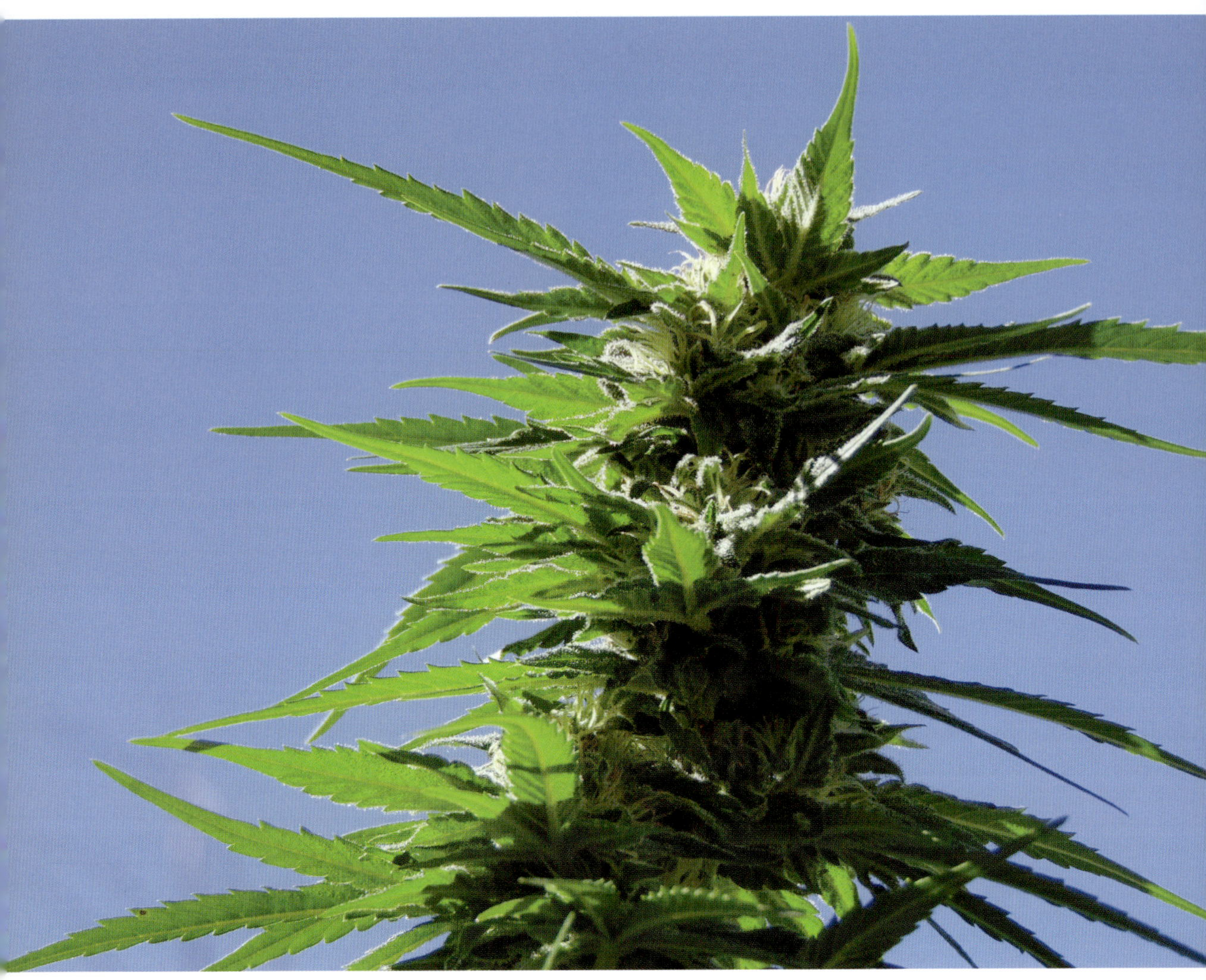

AK-47

above—Outdoor AK-47 cola in full sun. It's not my plant, but I couldn't pass up the opportunity to see what I could do with her. As it turns out, there were many options.

Foxy Lady

following page—I believe this one speaks for itself. I will only add that I don't want you to miss the cute little fox face. I'm sure you will find it now.

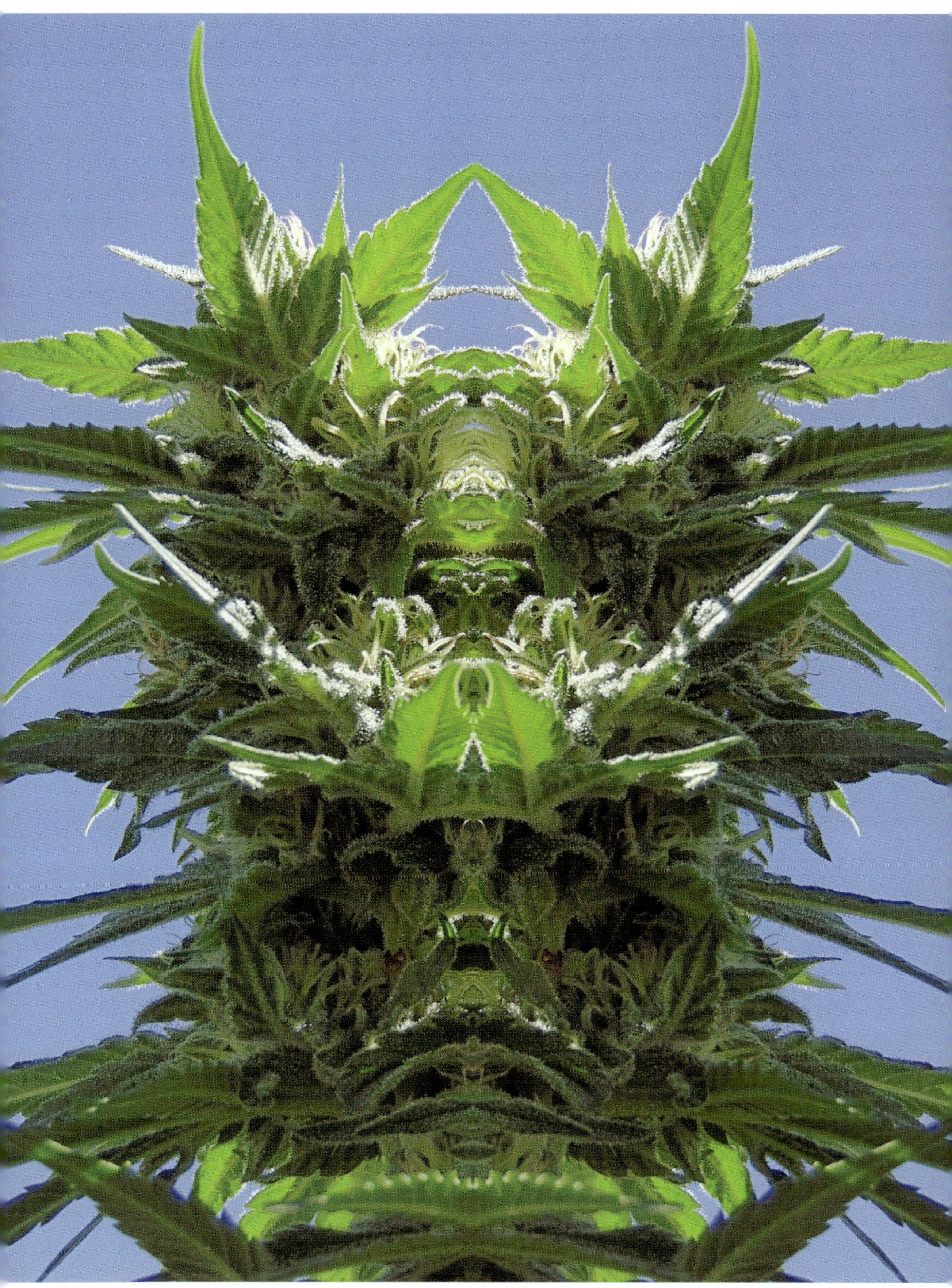

Twelve Petals

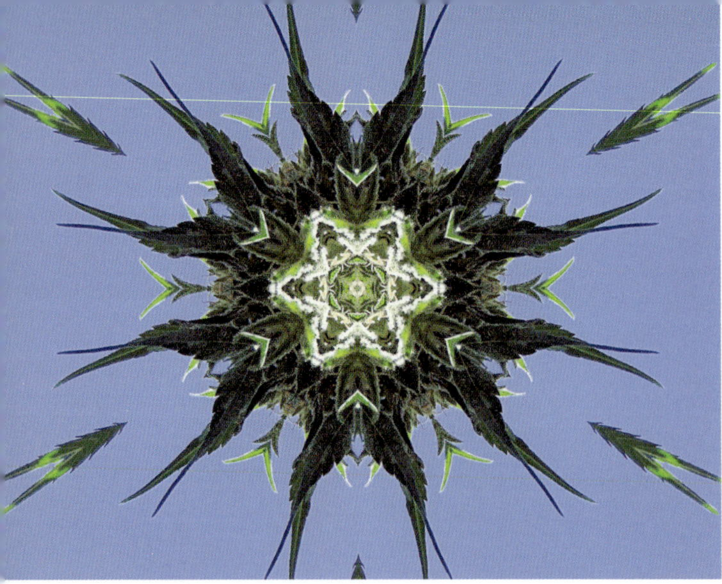

top—This twelve-petal AK-47 against the blue sky looks really sweet. Very different. I left the outer set of leaves in the image for this one to show what the clone feature can do.

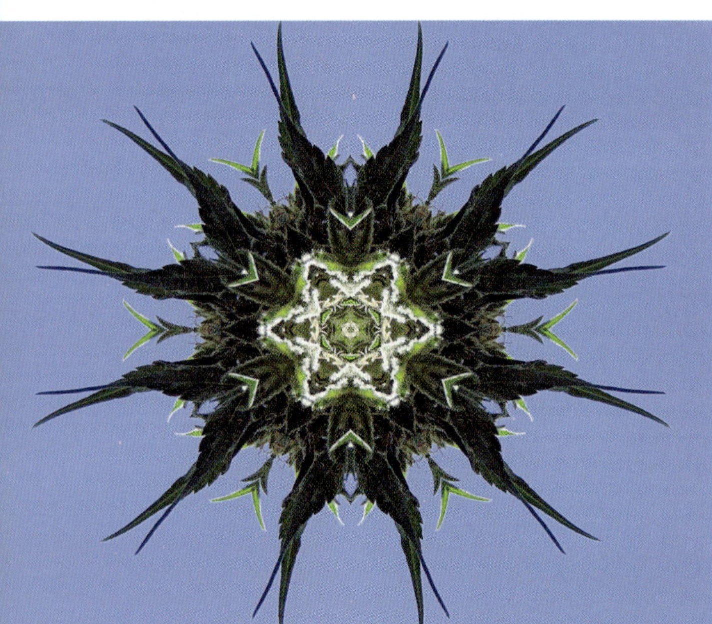

bottom—The outer set of leaves is gone. Cloning an area can be tricky. In this case, it was pretty easy to get good coverage because the blue is so solid. I can adjust the size of the brush for different scenarios. This image allowed for a large swath to be covered at one time. Brush size starts at 1 pixel, so you can really go nuts if you want to spend the time, but there are programs that make these eliminations much easier.

Surprise!

following page—Starting at the bottom fifth of the image, I see a being on top of the leaves. The sun causes his shadow to fall onto the leaves, and his head appears between them. The look on his face seems to indicate he was surprised to see me walk up to him. There are other cool beings on the way up, and there's another canna-bird at the top.

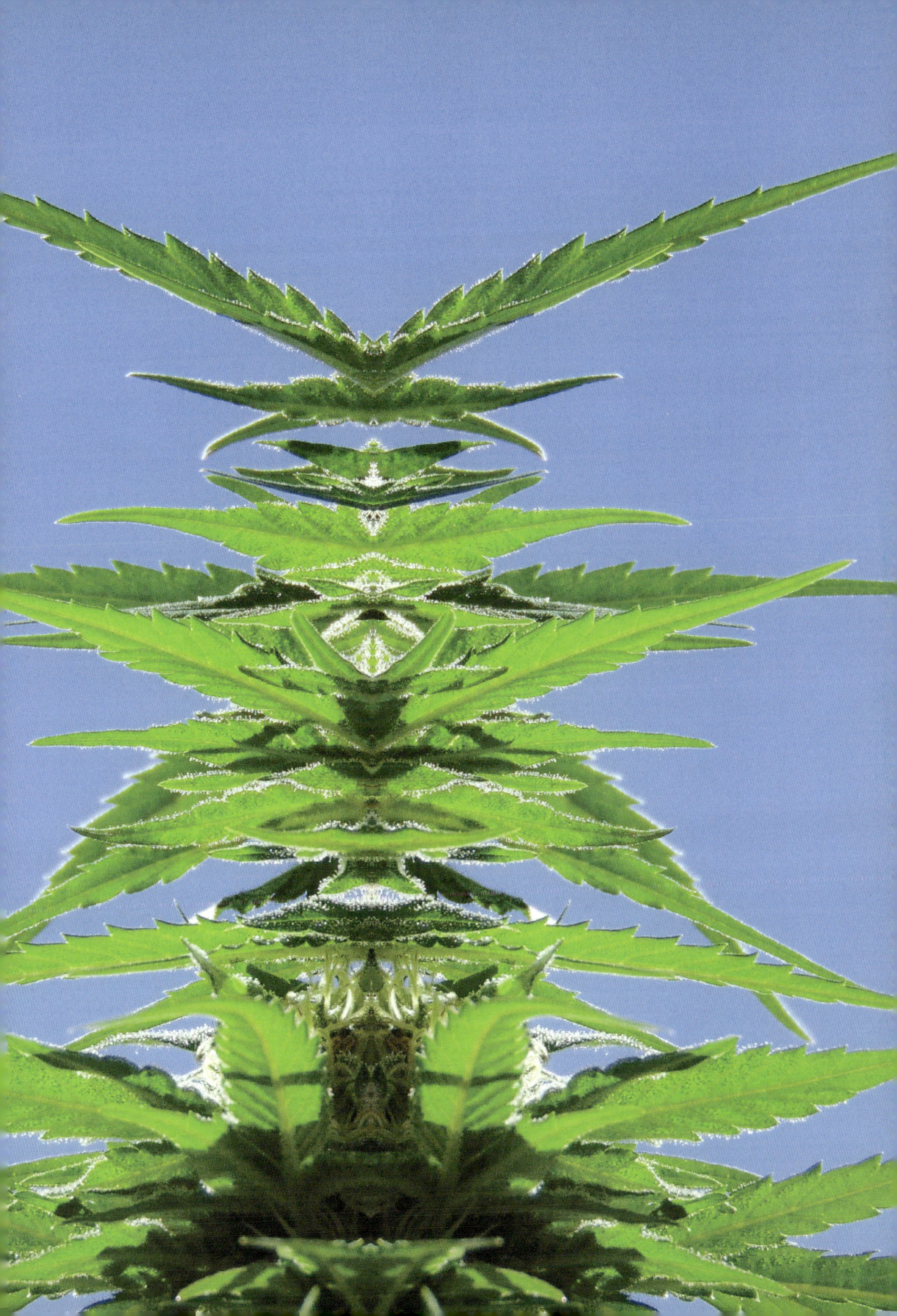

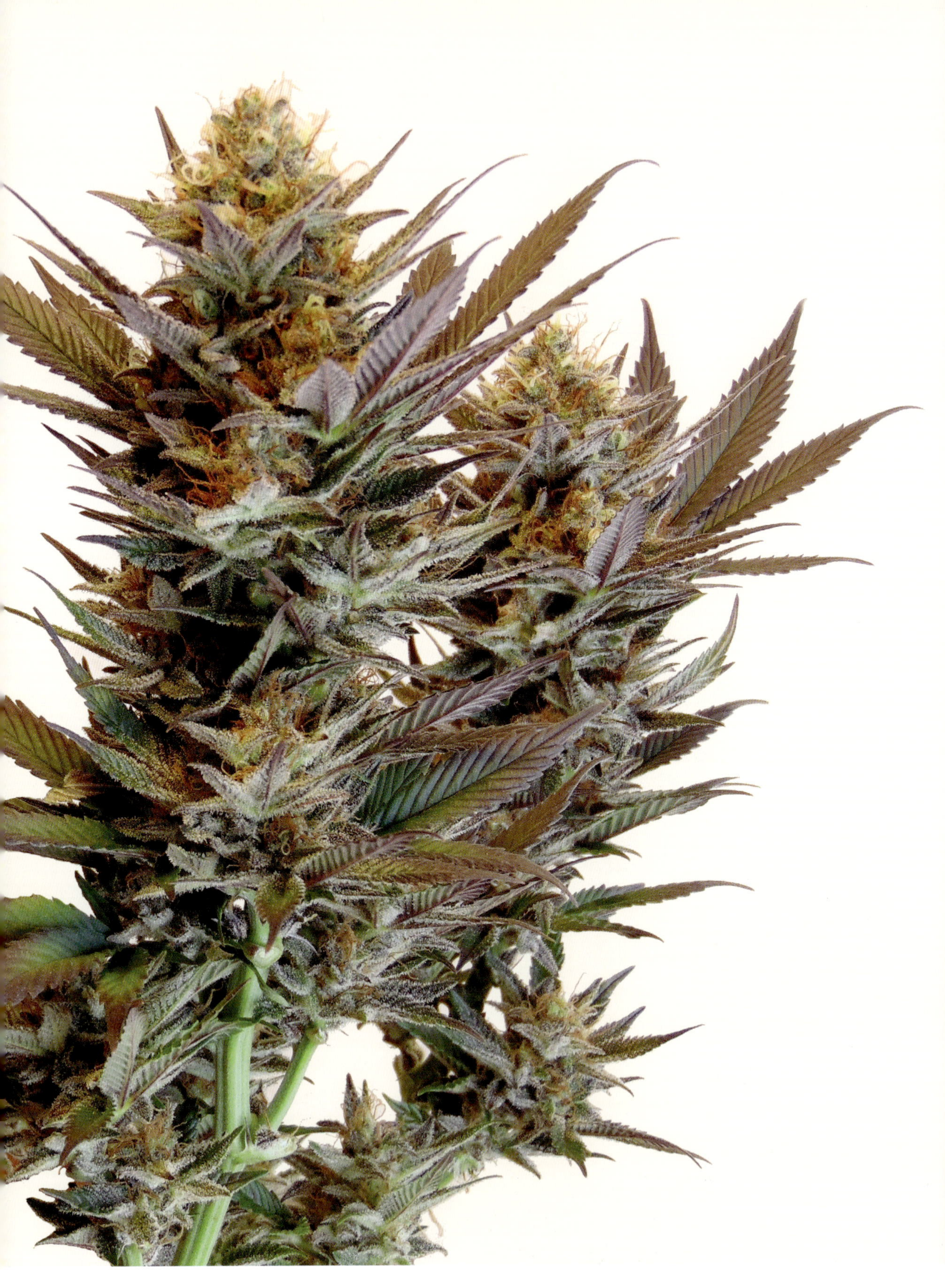

Indica Cross Series

previous page—This is the original indica cross image. I shot this with the intent of producing a nice cover image for a magazine. I ended up playing with it and made a number of interesting mash-ups.

below—There are two dogs with butterflies on their noses. The one near the top is very surprised!

page 88—A piggyback ride—or is it buds playing leap frog? I'm not sure.

page 89—Here's the same image, this time, with a purple background. I think I like this one best.

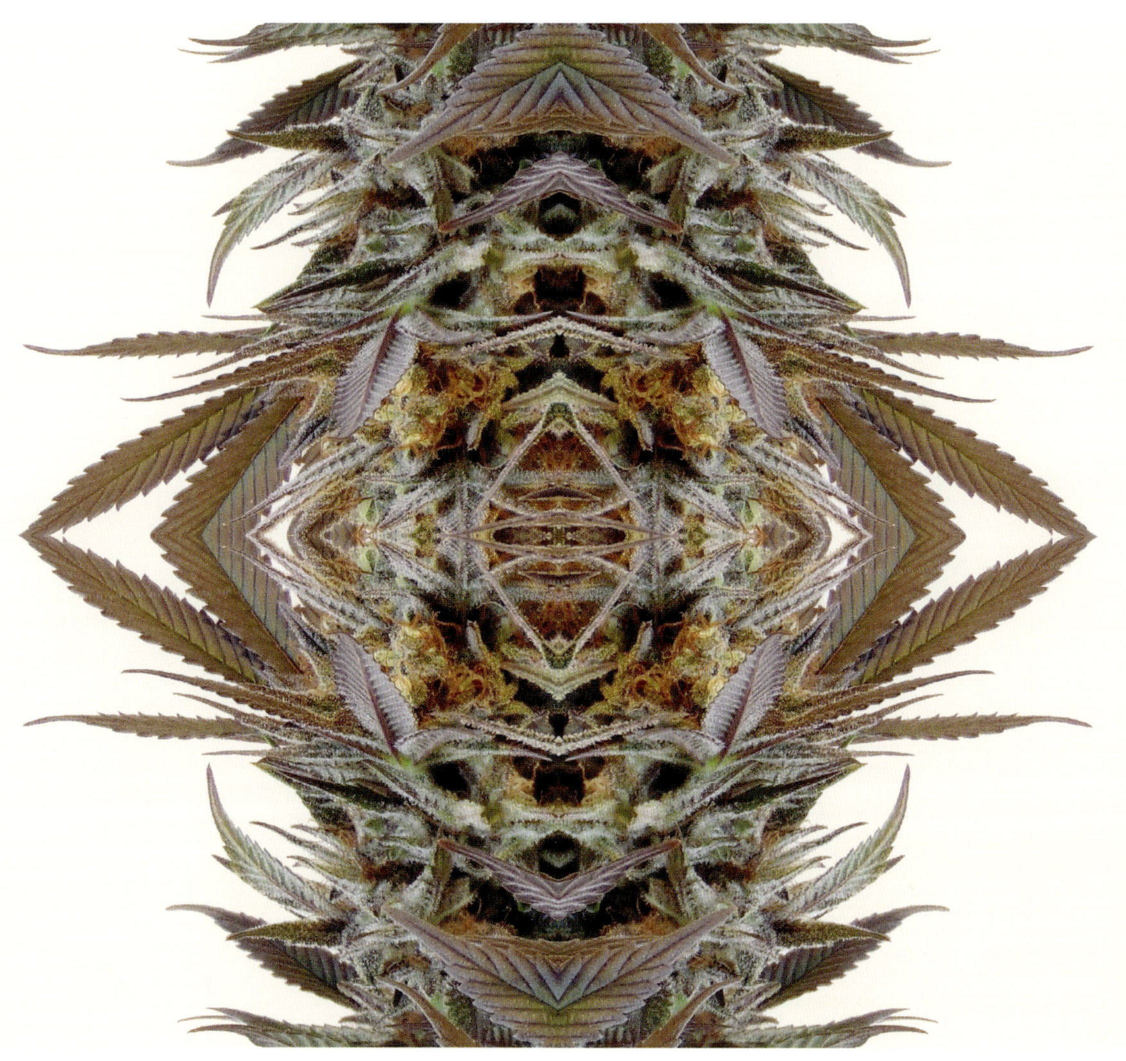

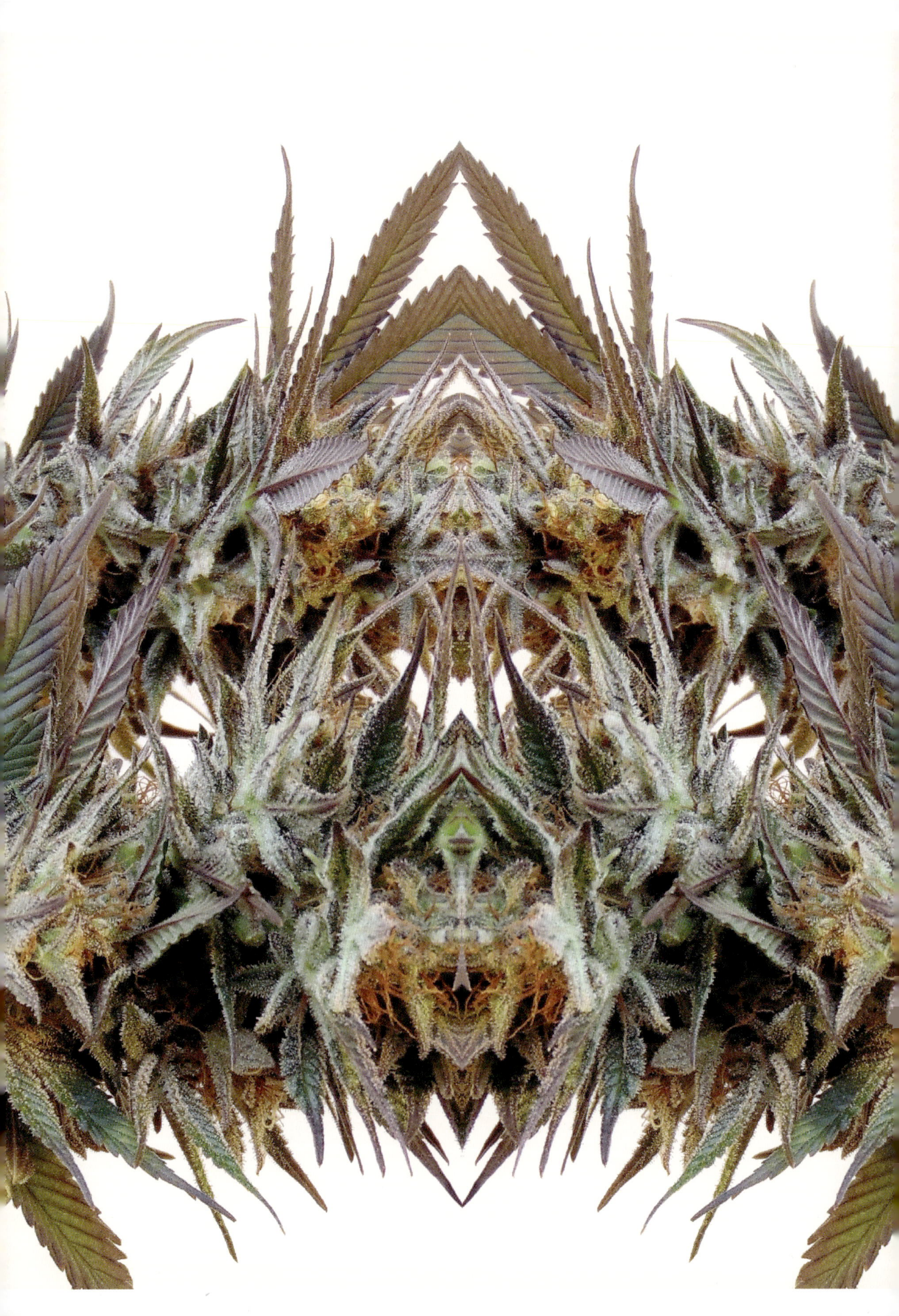

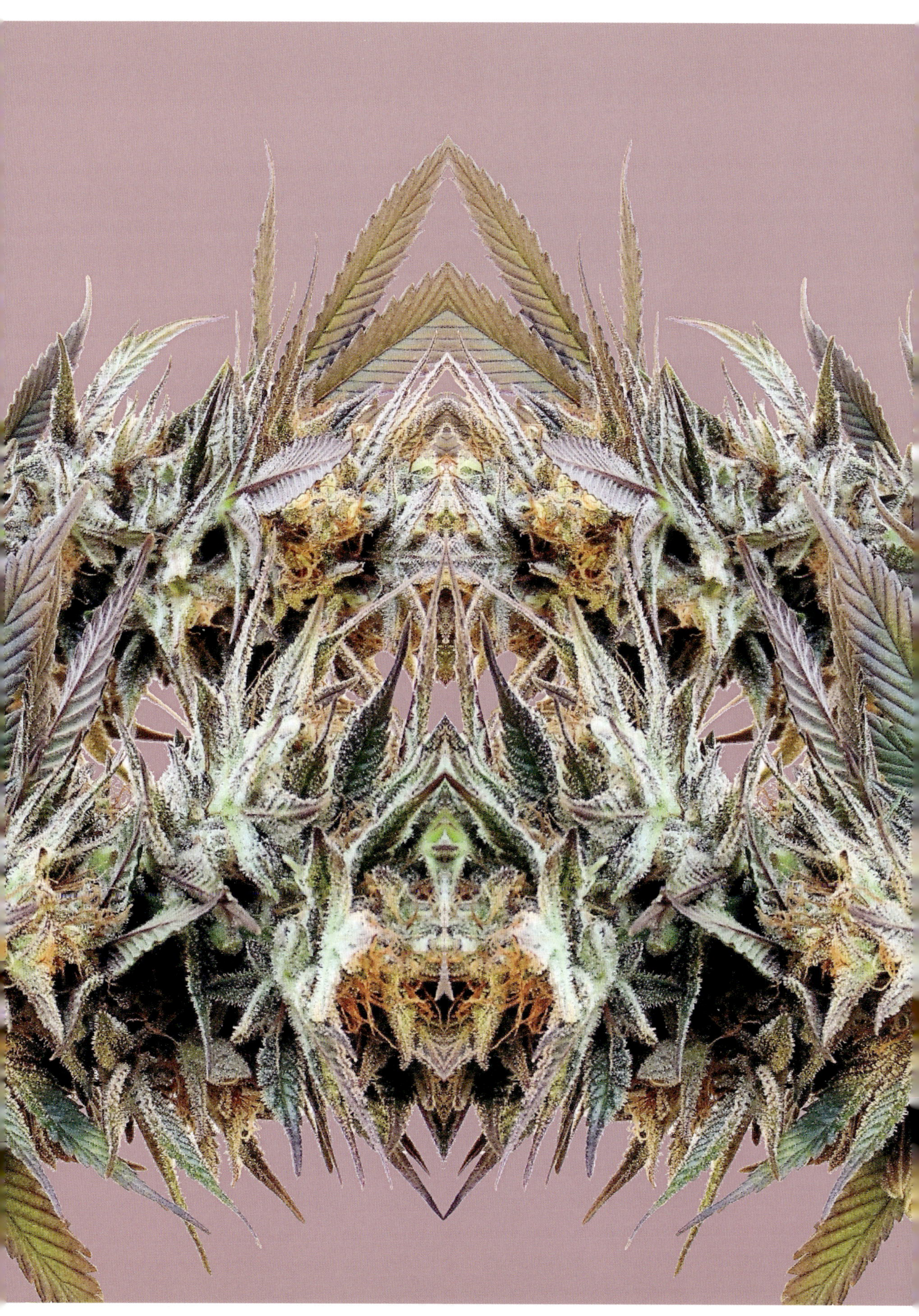

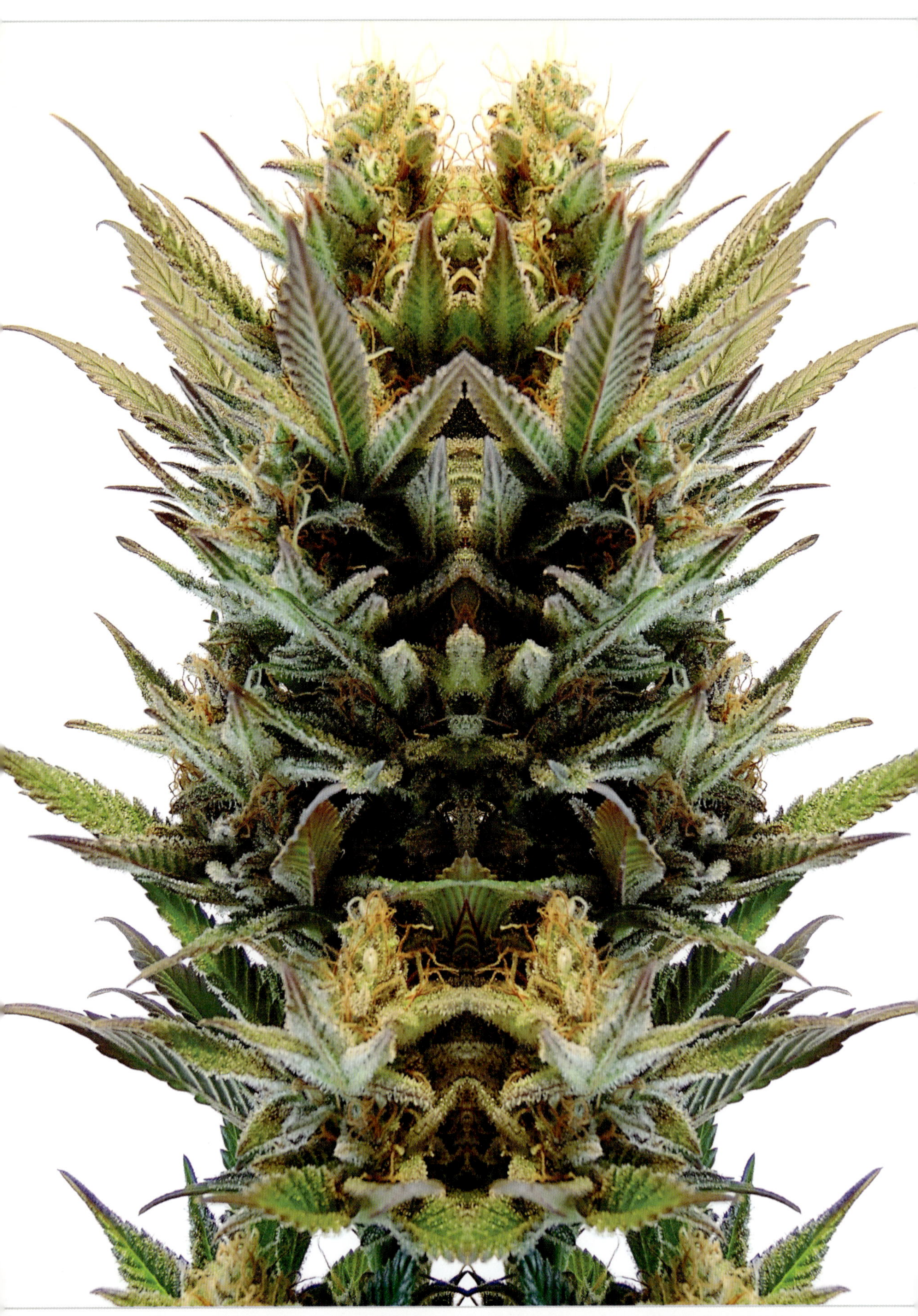

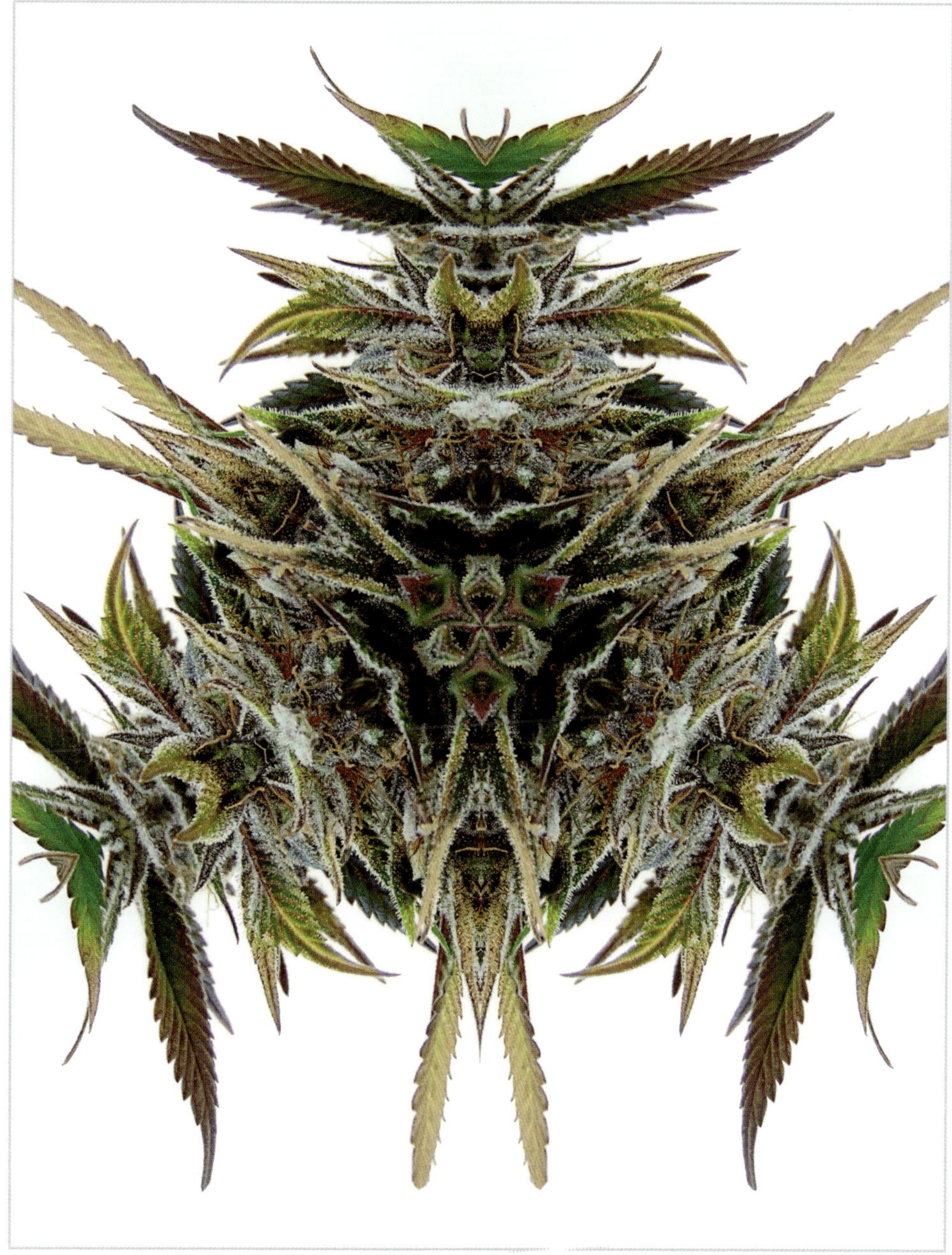

Building Blocks

previous page—Here's another image that I recommend viewing from six feet away. Close up, I really like the guy behind a table playing with building blocks; you'll see him at the upper part of the bottom third of the image. It looks as if he is staring intently at the little structure he has built.

Rife with Life

above—What do you see? I see more of those canna-birds. I also see a squirrel. You may also see a being with long ears and horns like a bison!

The Flock

below—More birds! Plus, when you view the image as a whole, it appears as if this being is looks cross-eyed and surprised as he tries to figure out where his nose went.

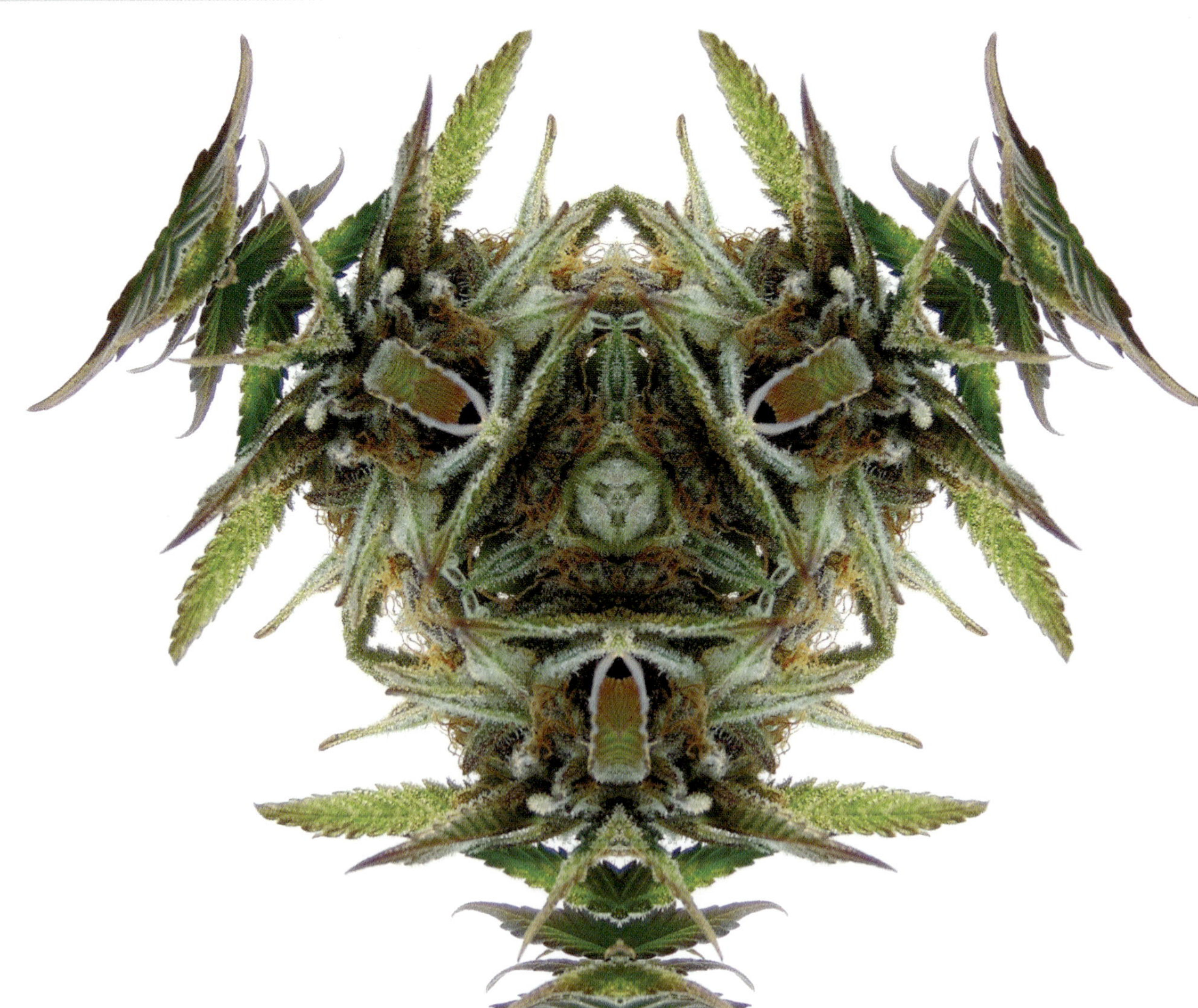

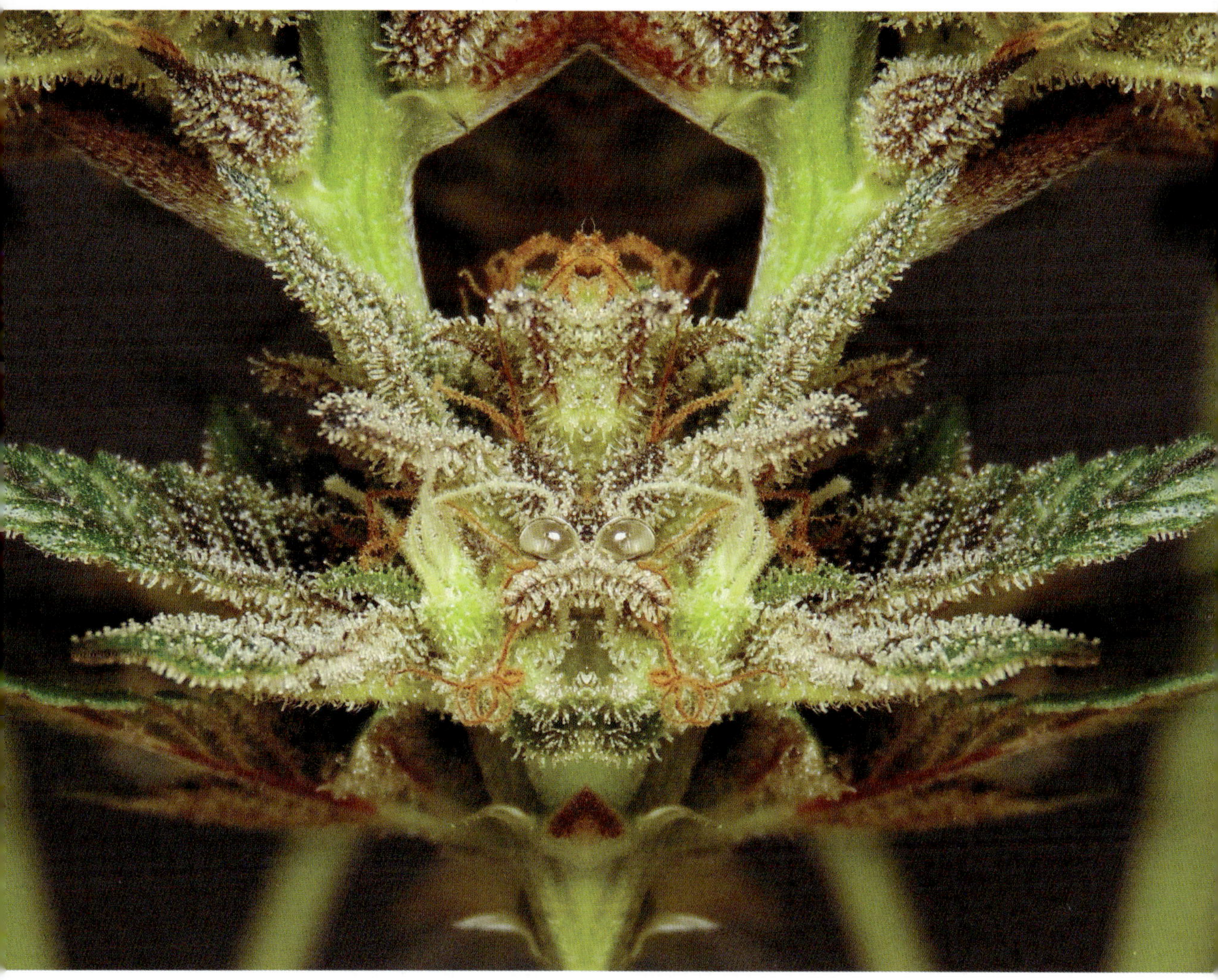

Whoa!

above—The cannabis fly trap? Canna-fish? Sure, I'll have a can of fish! Sorry, I couldn't resist. This bug-eyed creature made me say *whoa* when I mirrored it. Those googly eyes of sugar helped transform the image into something special. The eyes led me to see the trichome-packed upper lip, then a mouth that shows depth. Finally, the green lower jaw completed the face.

Seedy Delivery

top—I simply spread out some seeds on a plate and formed a half of a heart with my hands. It did take a while to flatten them out and keep reshaping it, but it was worth the effort, especially since I knew I didn't have to do the other side—I could just mirror it.

bottom—The heart turned out really well. In postproduction, I dumped brown around it to fill in the area. Unfortunately, there were little gaps along the outside of the heart. I used the clone tool to fill in the gaps between every seed on the outer edge of the heart to make this image work. There are even faces down the middle!

following page—I love mandalas, and I just had to find a good one for these seeds. This image shows twenty petals, and there are many faces to be seen in the seeds.

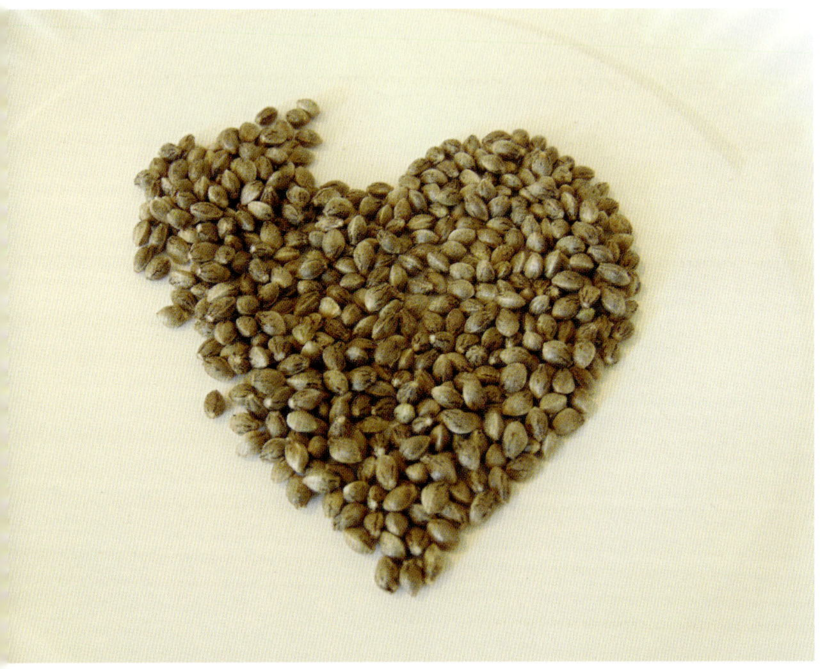

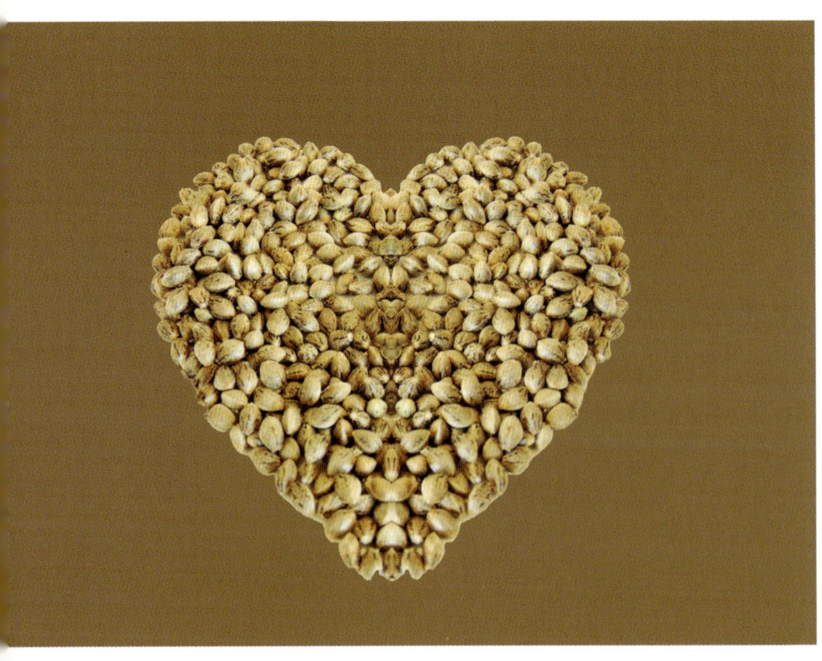

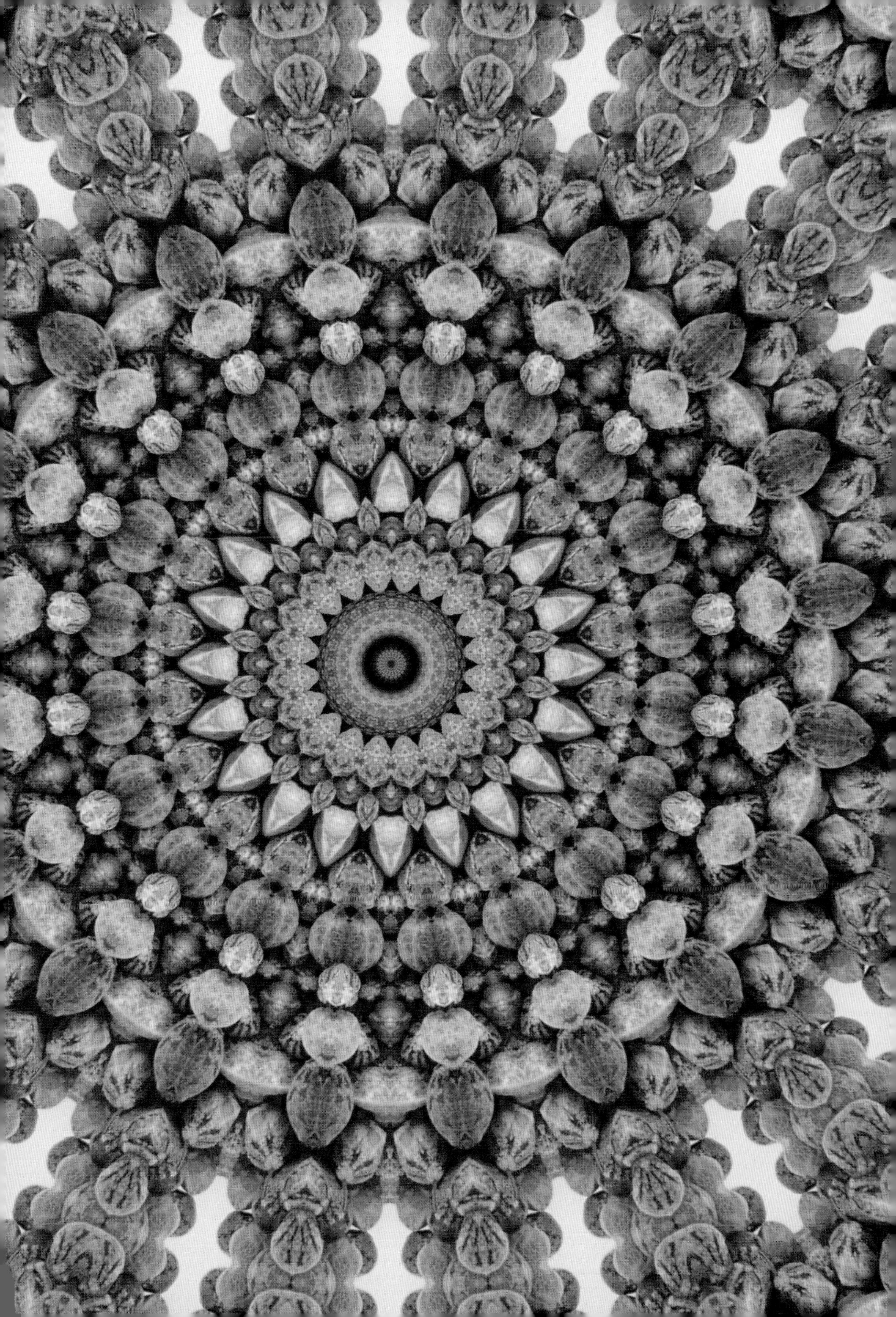

Evergreen

top—I placed a couple of the dry indica buds in a pine tree just to see what would happen when I ran it through the post-processing gamut. You never know!

bottom—I love what happened in this six-petal mandala. The buds are still recognizable, forming a circular shape. There are faces everywhere. Look closely, and you can see a circle of beings, arm in arm, gazing up at you. This mostly mature indica loved going outdoors for a shot of sunshine. The purple was heavy on this crossbreed, and even the leaves have a ton of glands.

following page—Another variation.

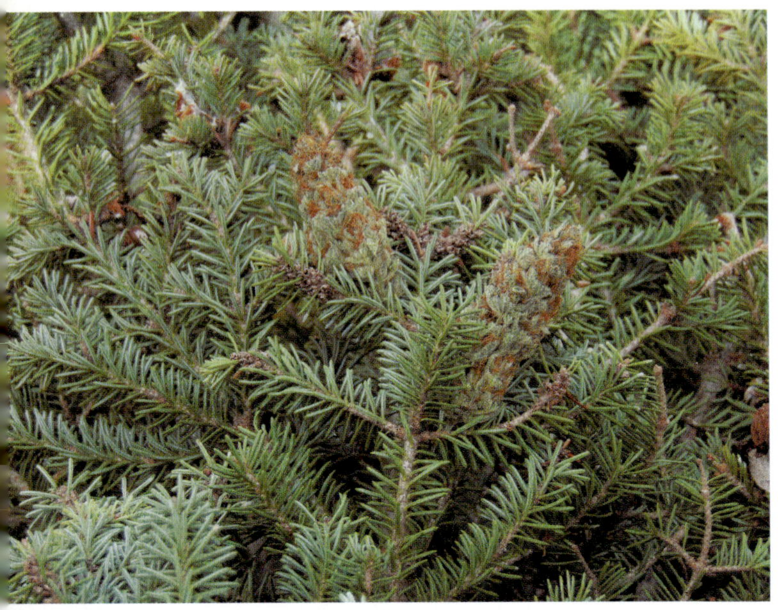

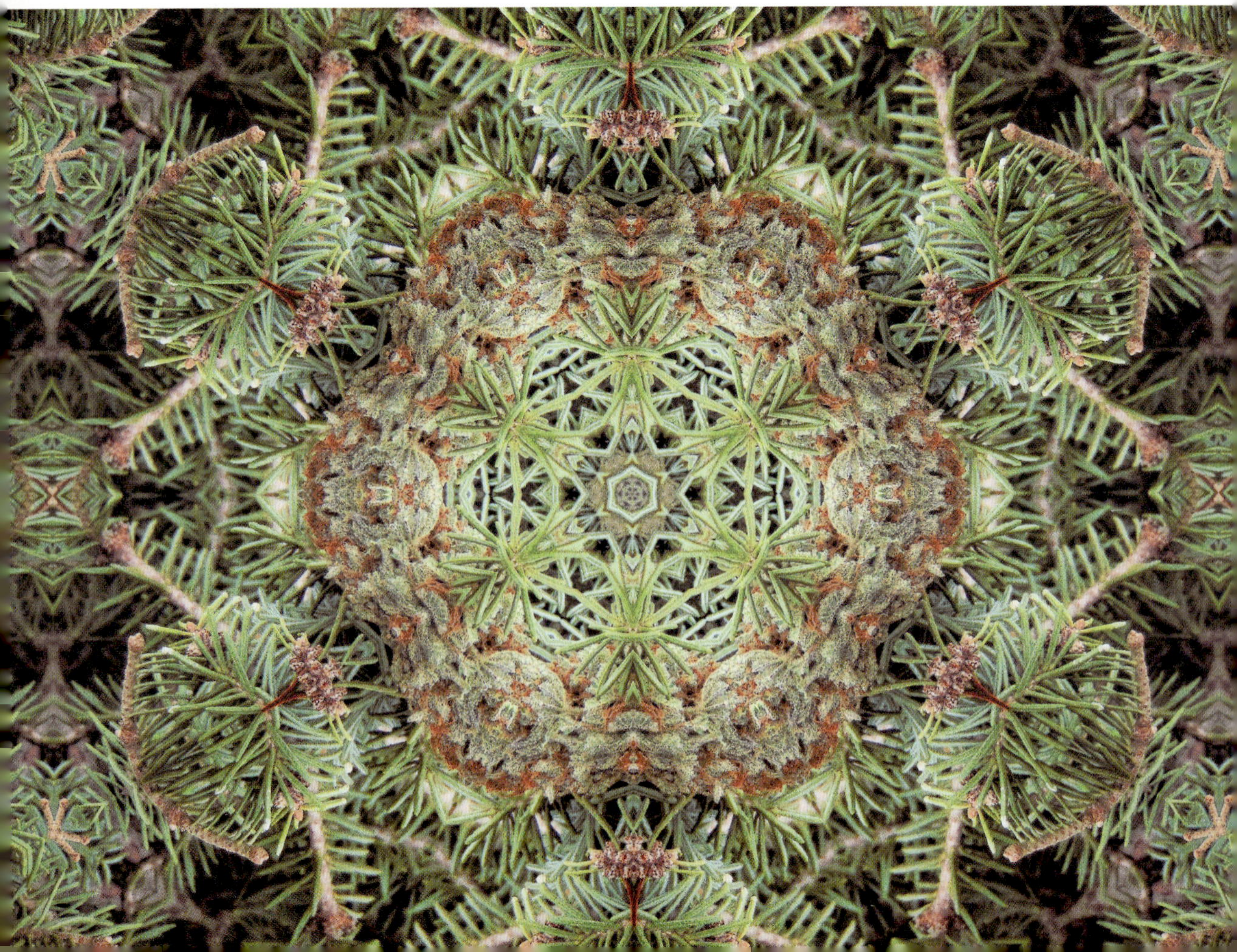

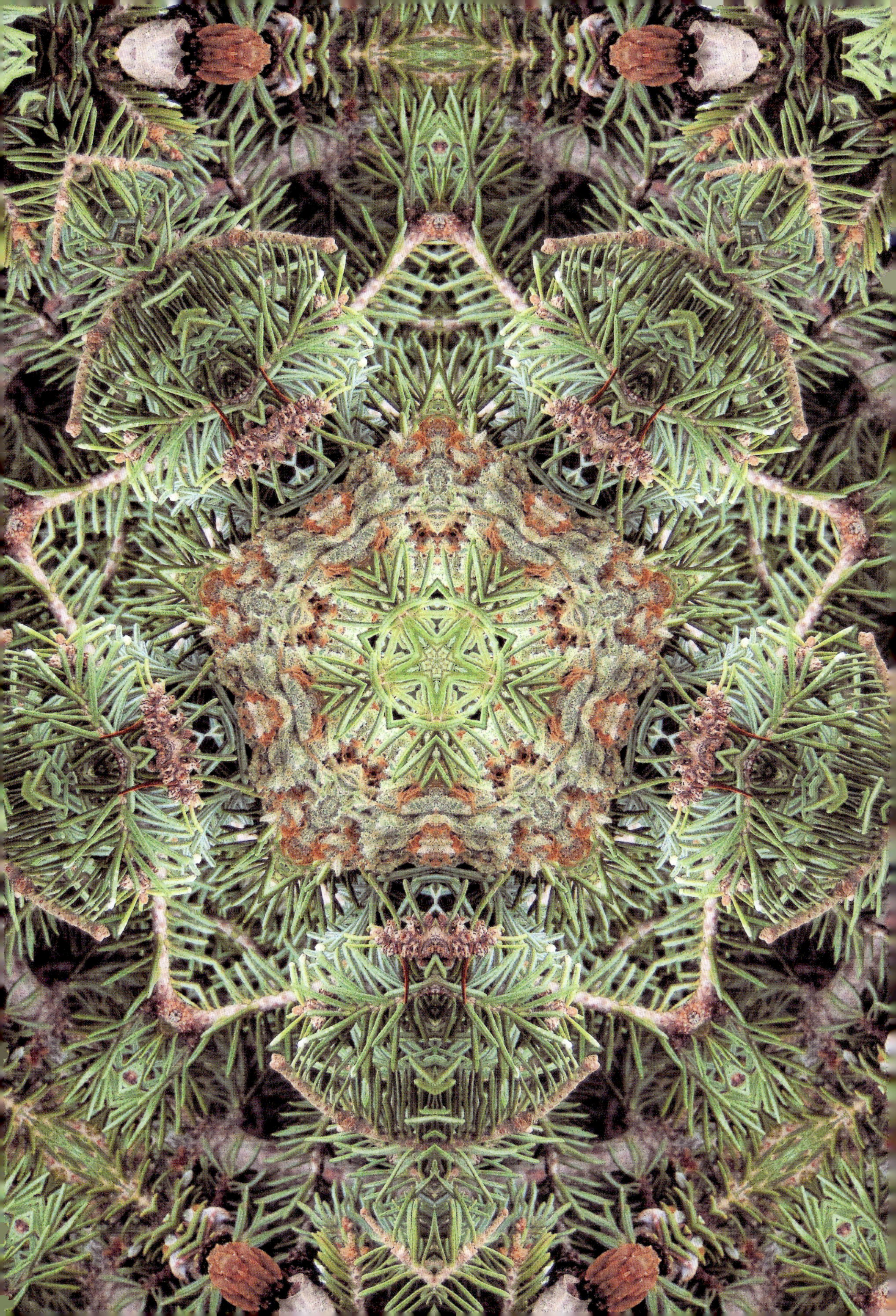

Starting Point

top—I brought this Blue Dream plant outside in the morning and took a few images. This is

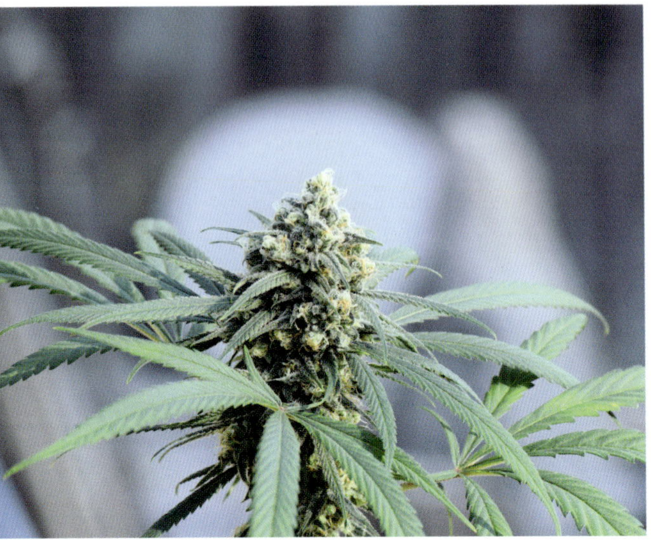

the cropped original. This plant is about ten days away from being just right to harvest.

Dreaming

bottom—This one was cropped closer and mirrored to form a few faces, though there aren't as many as there are in most of my photos. The lighting and colors in this image were soothing to my eyes, especially after staring at the computer for so long!

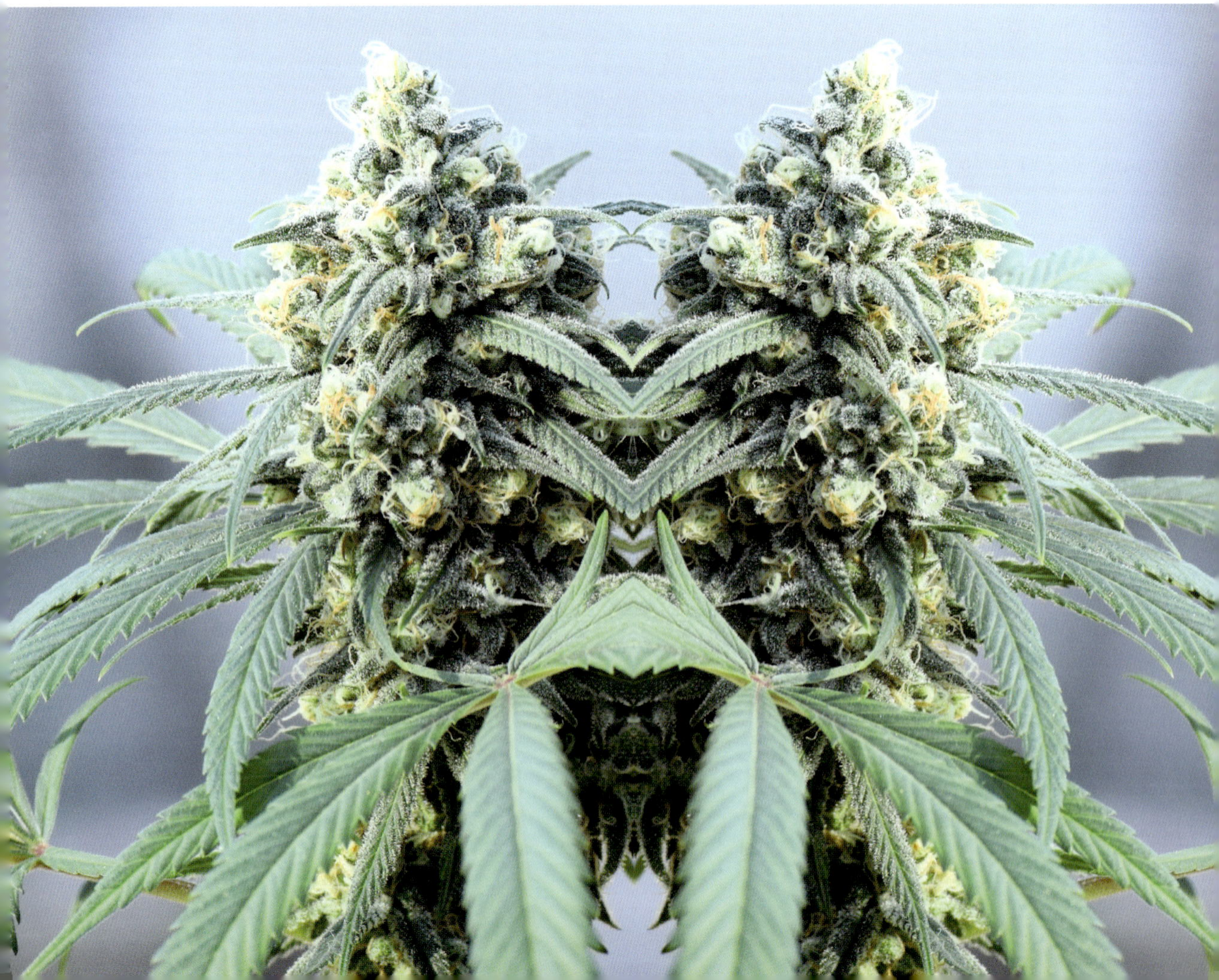

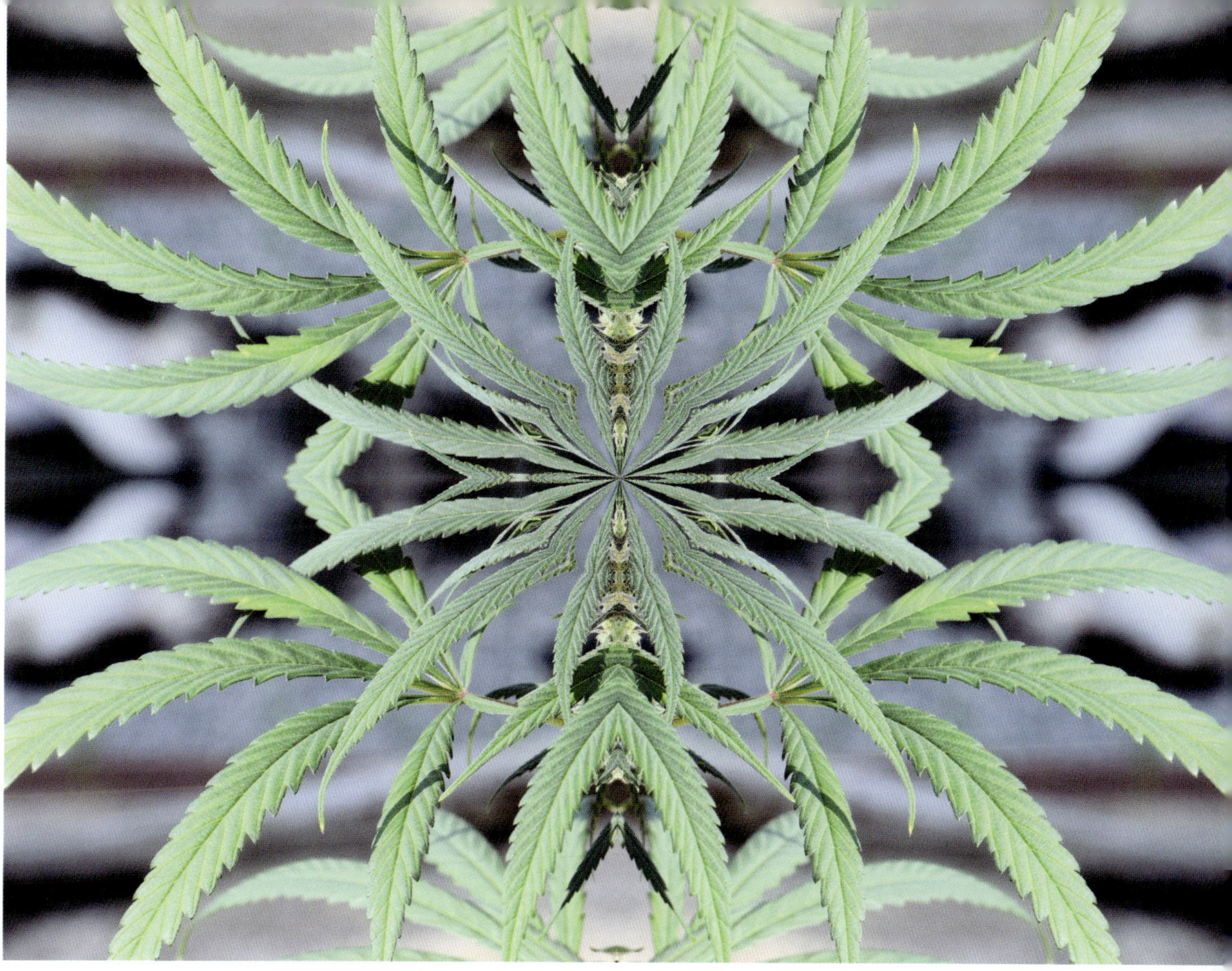

Leaf Play

top—It doesn't always have to be the buds that are right up front. These leaves come together to form a simple pattern that is easy on the eyes. The colors coordinate with the other images on this spread.

Montage

bottom—This completes a set of images. A grouping of images that complement one another look great as wall displays. Make your space stand out and celebrate the beautiful cannabis plant!

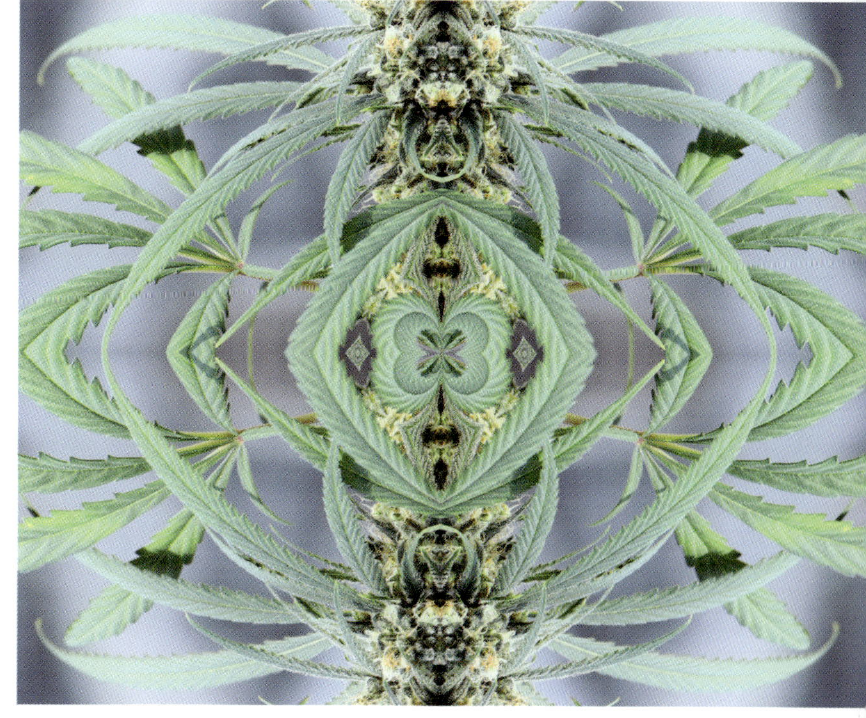

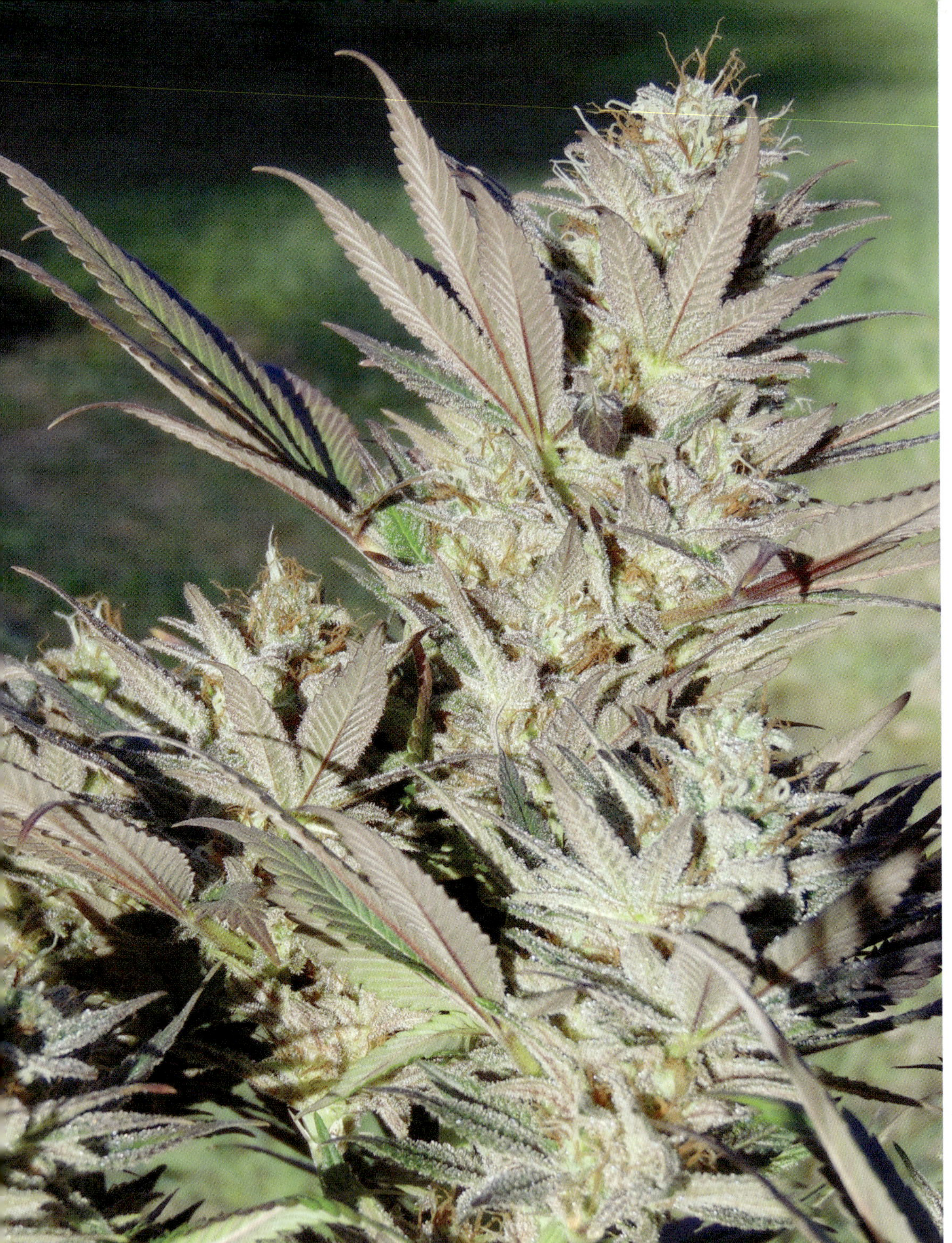

Fun in the Sun

above—This mostly mature indica loved going outdoors for a shot of sunshine. The purple was heavy on this crossbreed, and even the leaves have a ton of glands.

Mirror, Mirror

following page—Mirroring the previous image created this one. Go ahead and spend a minute or three looking around in there.

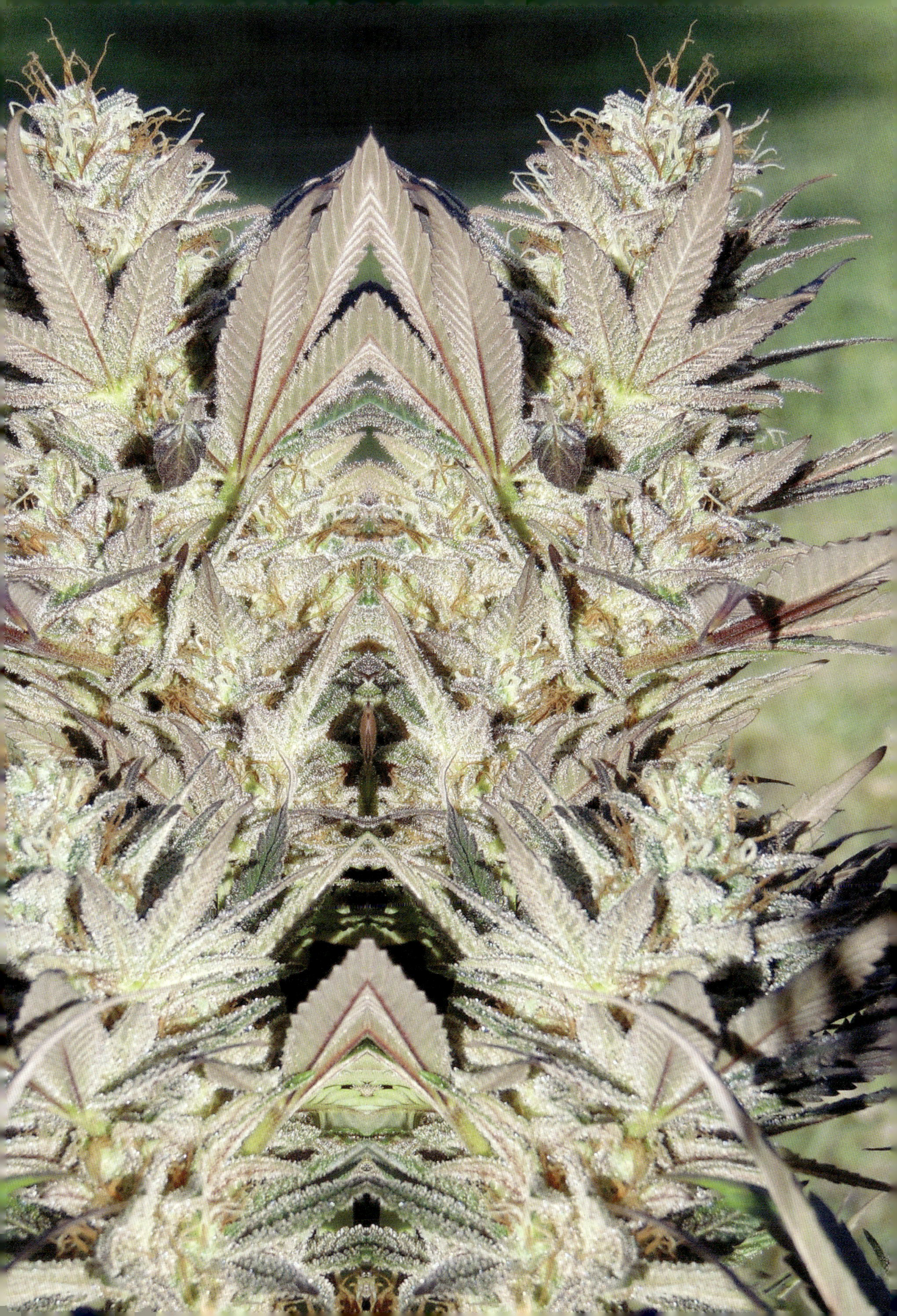

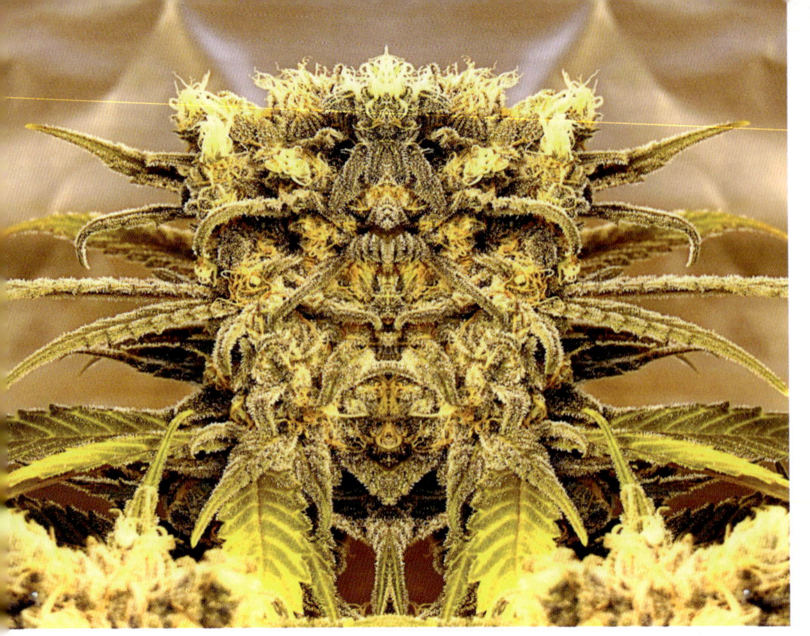

Friend

bottom—This is a very cool canna-being in a friend's garden. See the face dead center? It has oversized lips, and those eyes . . . they seem almost real. His arms are bent behind his back, and he wants to be sure you're a friend before you leave. Then again, if he knew he was in this book, he would know you are already a canna-buddy.

Fiber Art?

following page—When I made this image, I thought the pattern would be great for a rug. It seems to give off its own light.

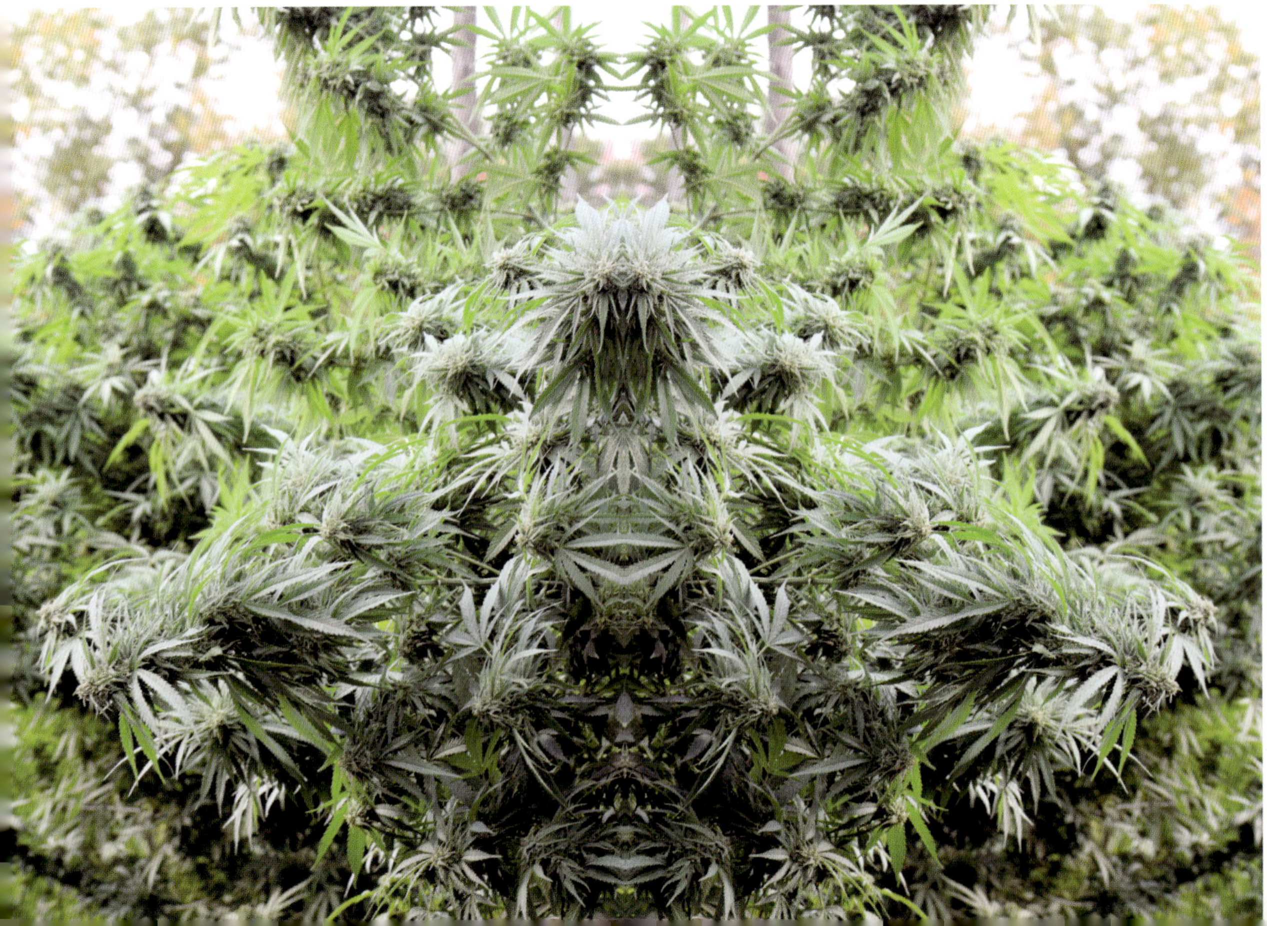

Serious Business

top—There's a lot going on here. When you check this out from a distance, and then view it close up, there's a big change, too. It's always best to try that approach with all the images, but doing so really makes a difference here. Don't make this guy angry. He might hulk out!

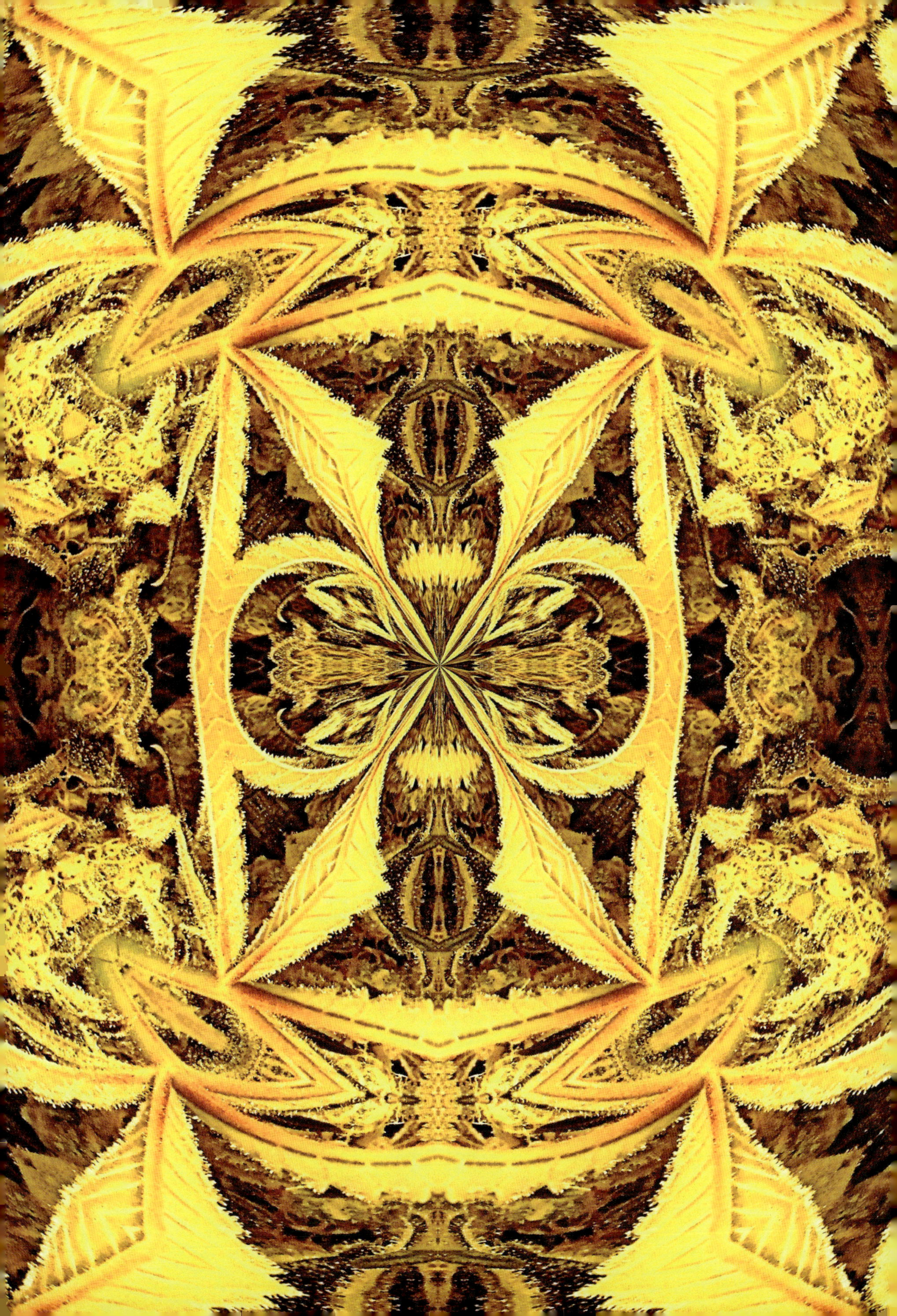

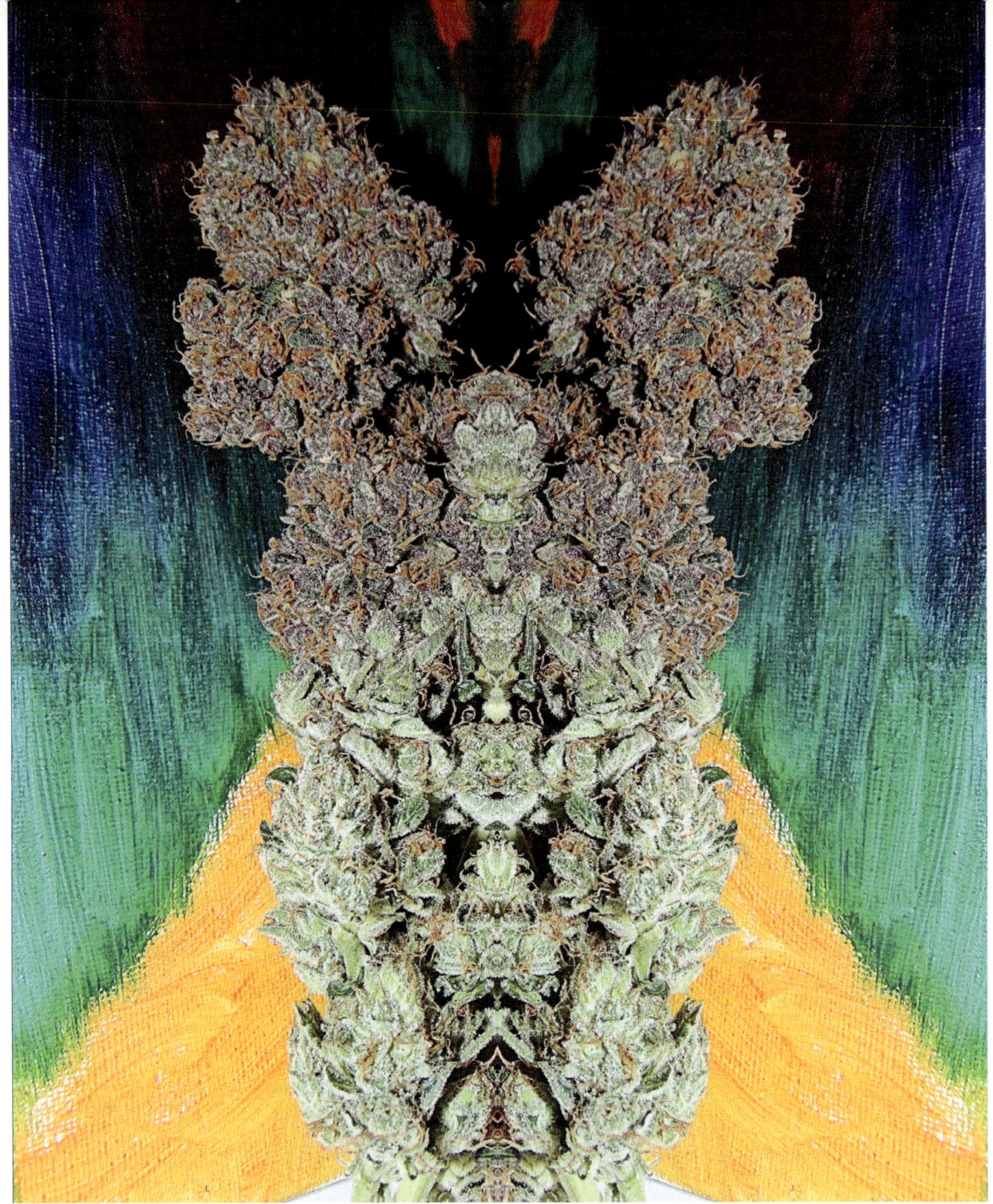

Rabbit

above—This image was made against a painted canvas. To create it, I opened some buds from the cola, inserted a different strain, and tucked them together for a tight fit. This is another "take a step back" image. It reminds me of a rabbit with a yellow jacket on.

Shadow Dance

following page—This image came about in a strange way. The sun was coming through the trees and filtered through a windowed door, then illuminated a small spot on the wall. There was a plant between the door and the wall, and it cast dancing shadows. Idea! My wife removed that plant while I grabbed a fresh leaf. She ducked down to hold it by the stem, and the shadow was cast. I mirrored the leaf, added a color twist, and the image was done.

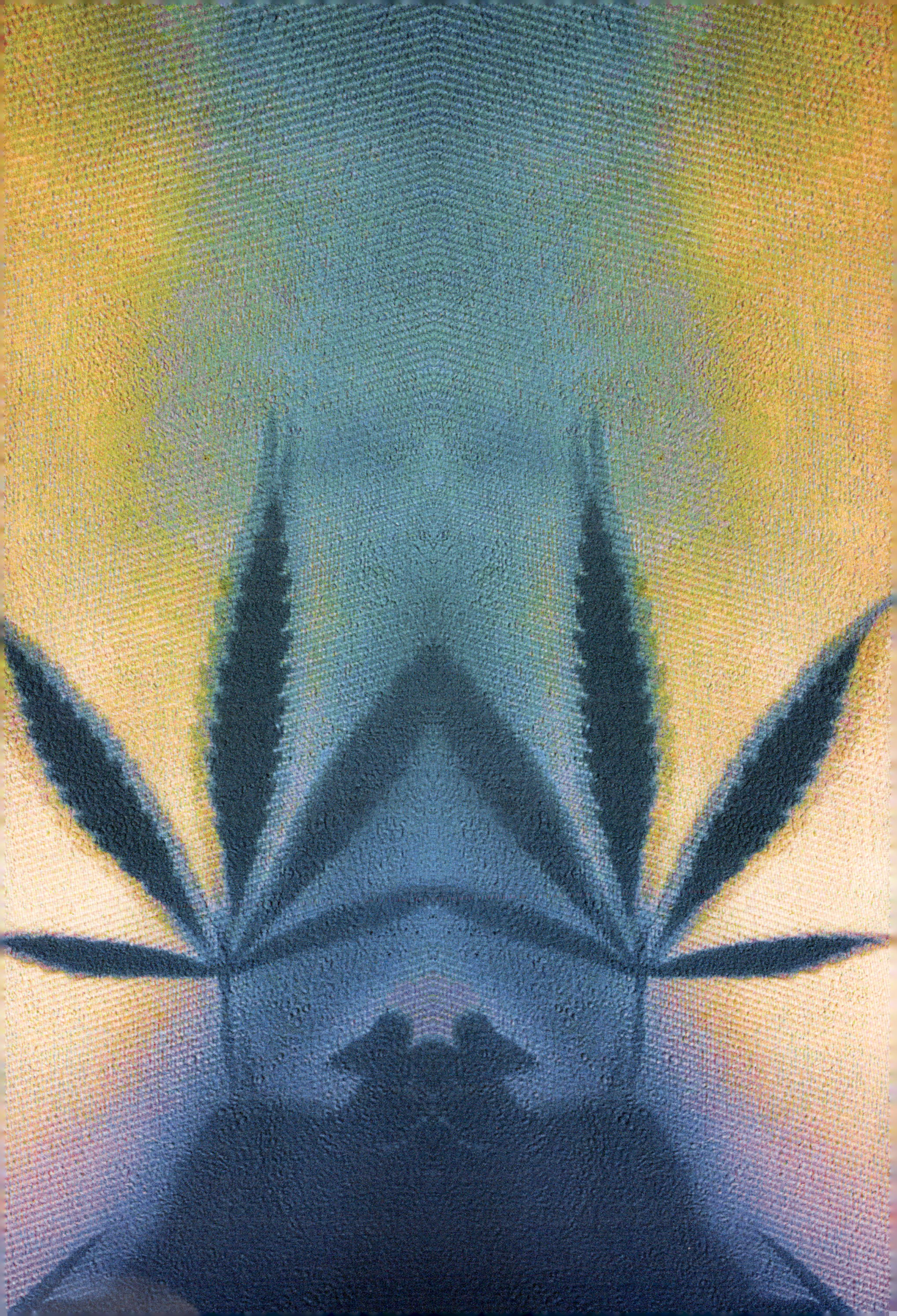

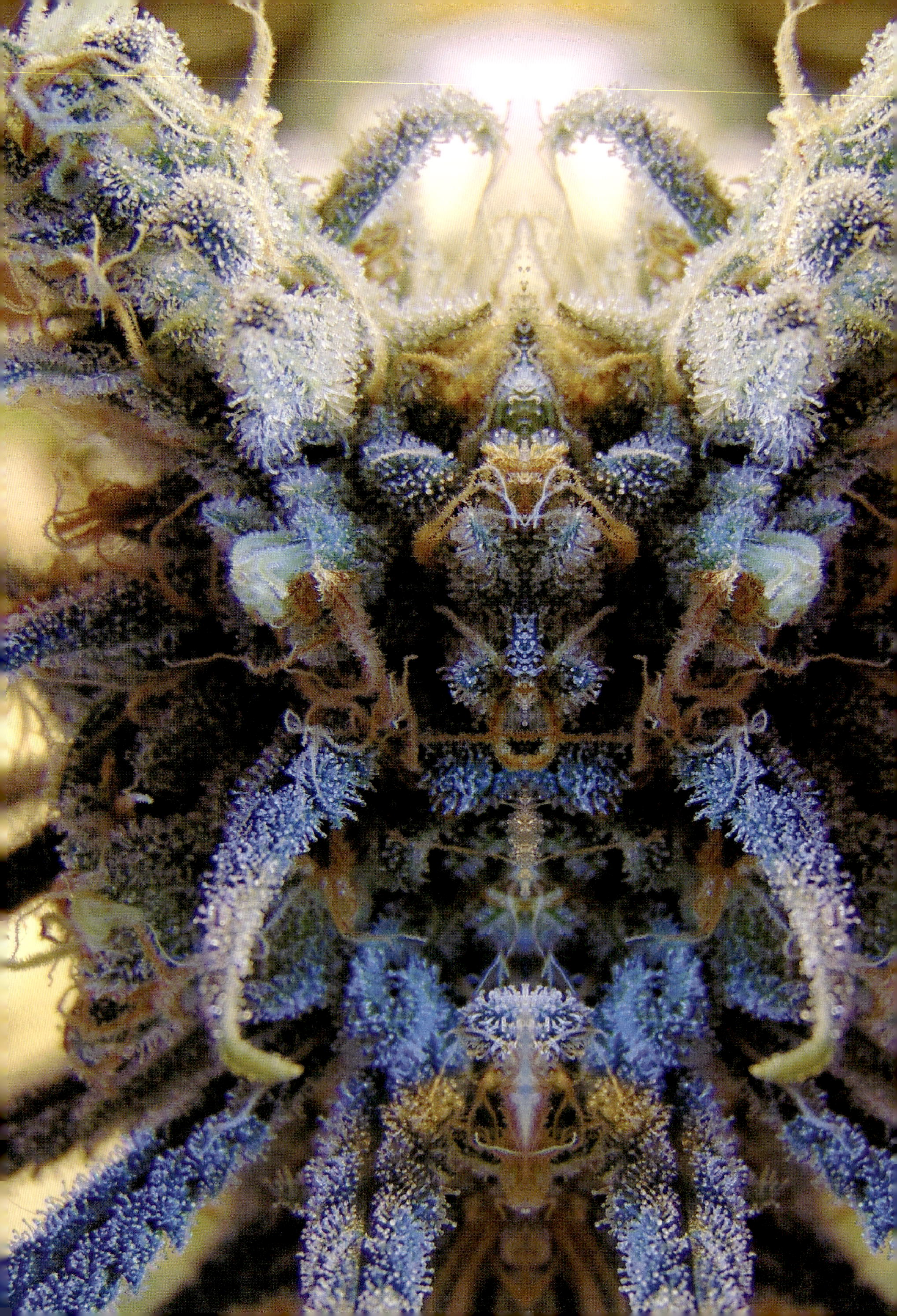

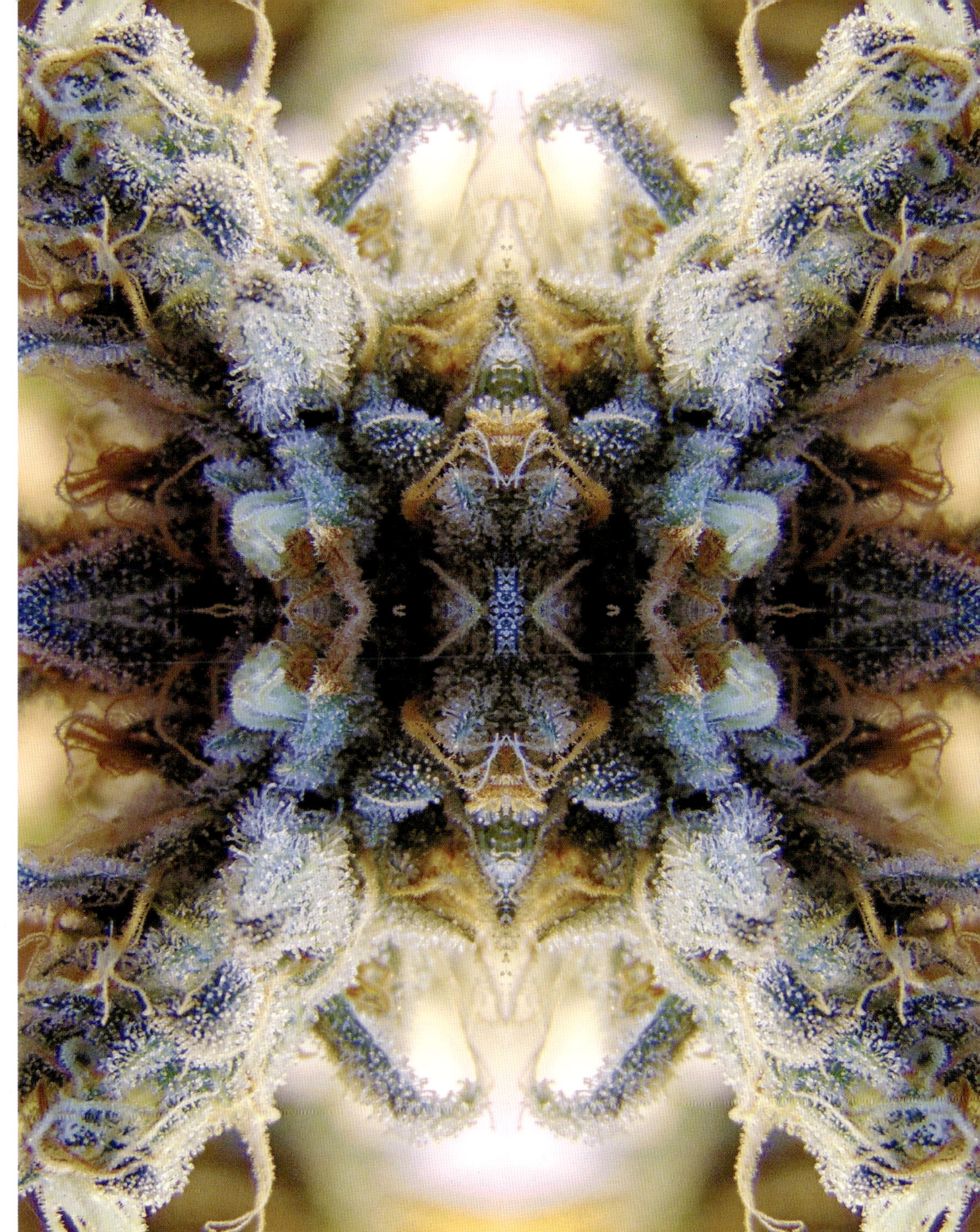

Flexing

previous page—Blue and gold go together like peanut butter and jelly, and there's no shortage of those colors here. This being is flexing its muscles and showing off his gear.

Another Take

above—I turned the image on its side and mirrored it again, and this was the result. This dude is absolutely built! I love the trichomes in both of these images.

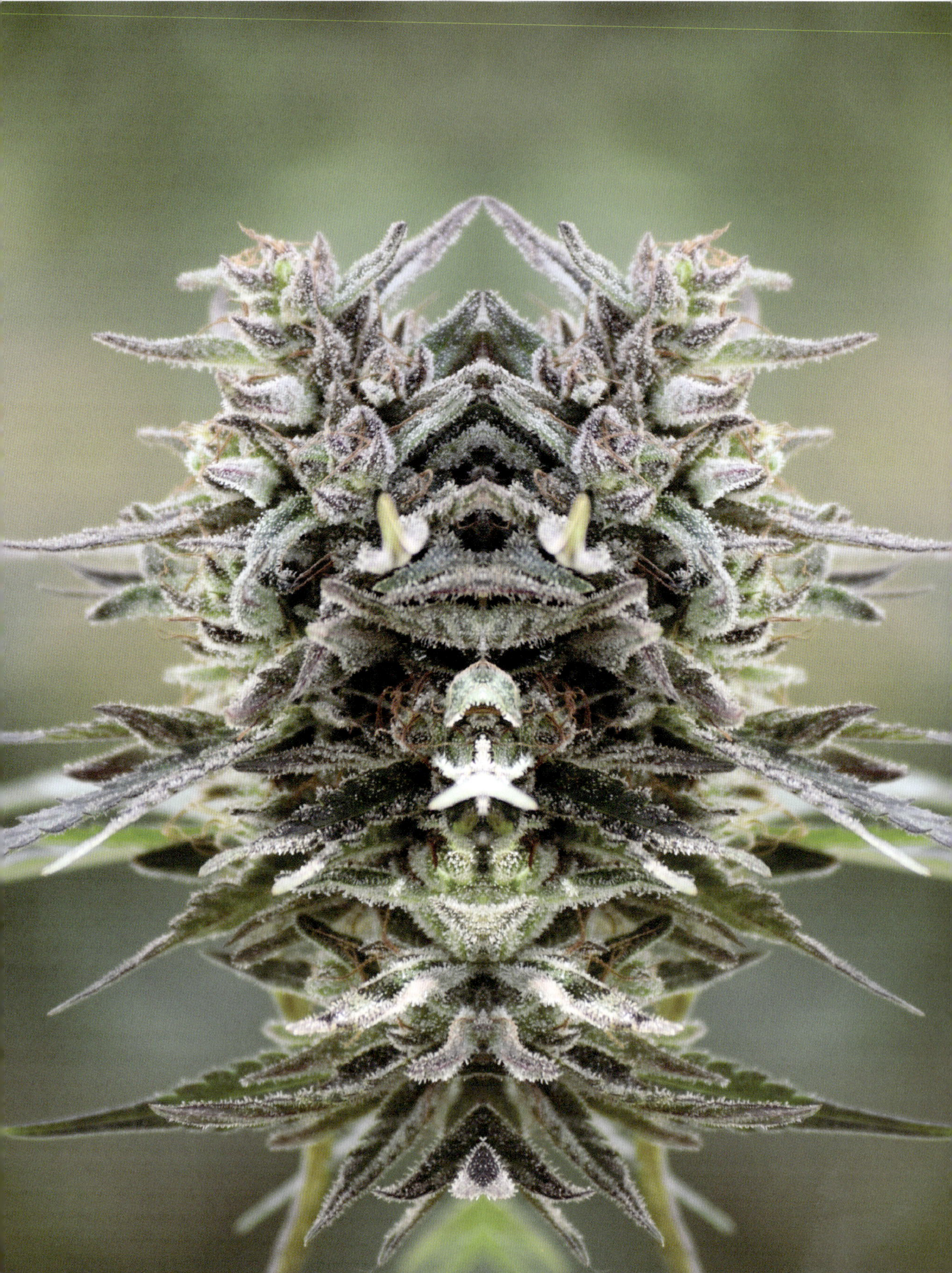

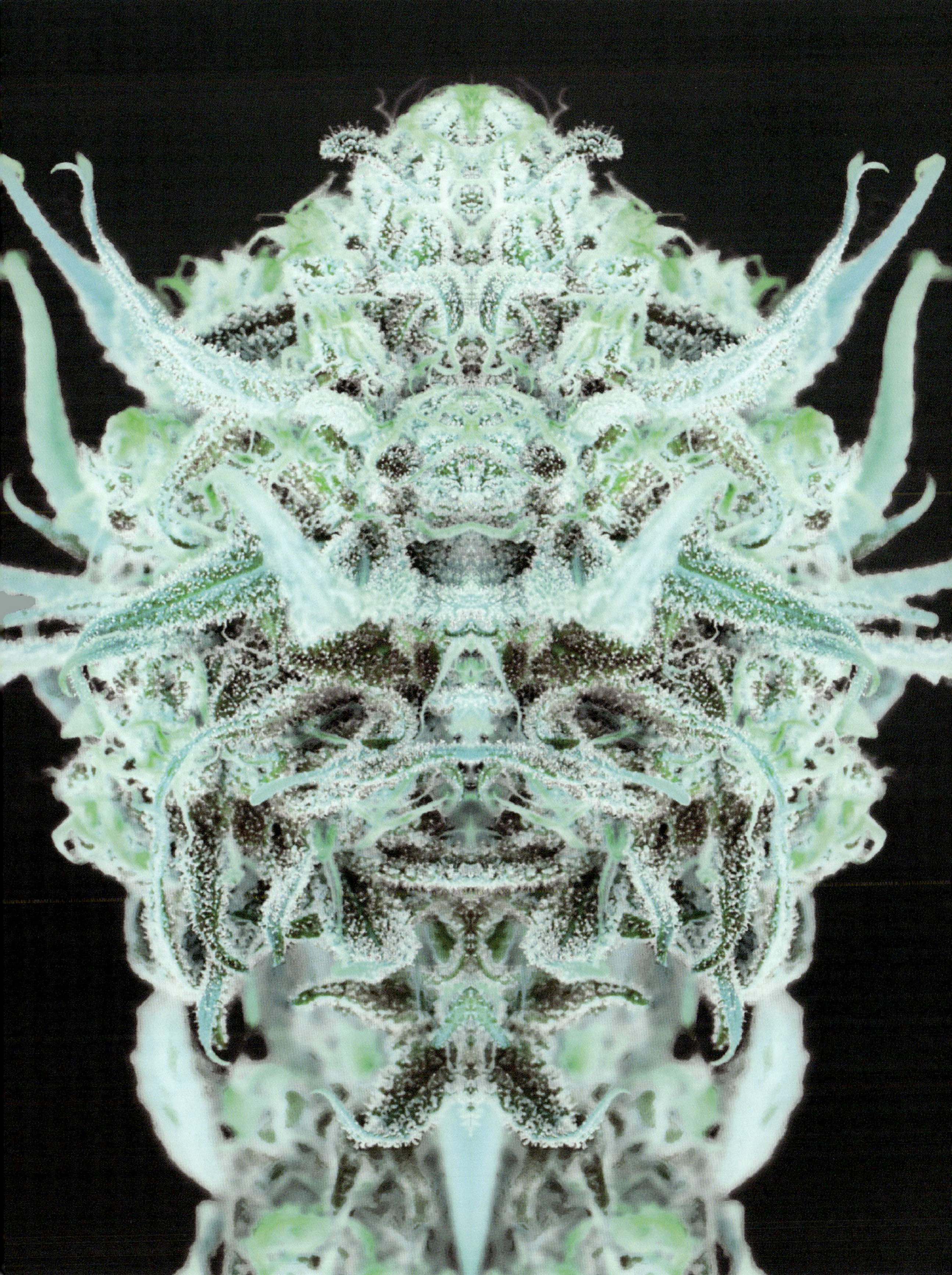

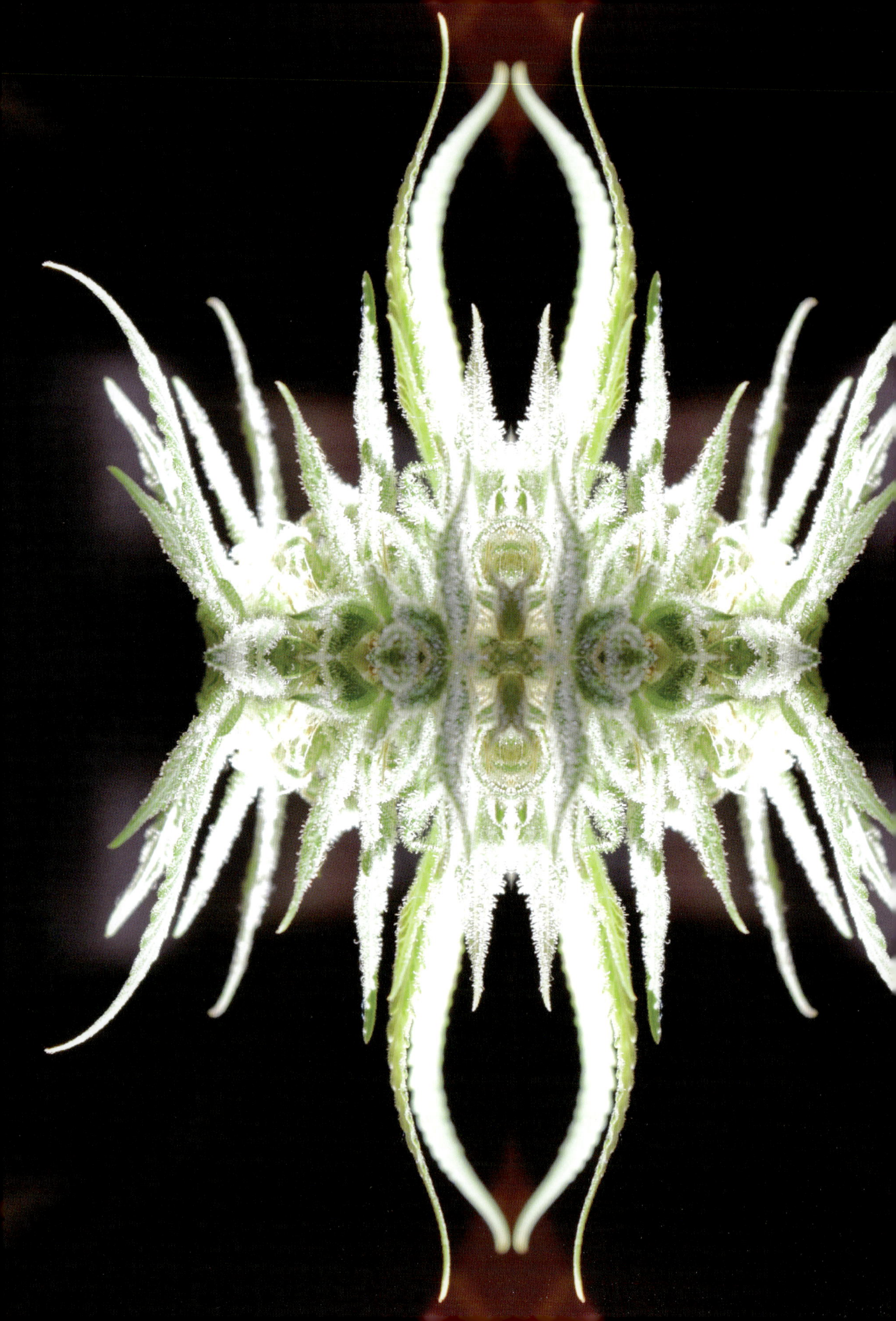

Sea Creatures

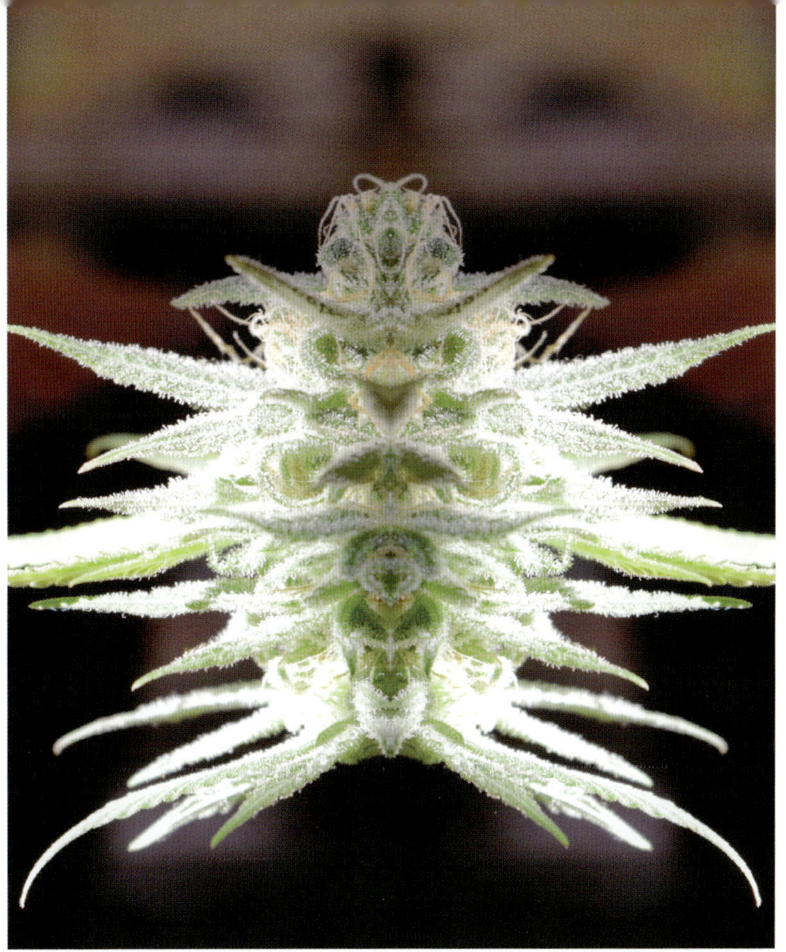

left—There's a little less detail to see in this image, but it stands out nevertheless. The original image was lit on the right side with a flashlight, so when I mirrored it, the cannabis was fully lit.

previous page—Again, turning it sideways and mirroring it created a different perspective from which to view this glowing sea creature.

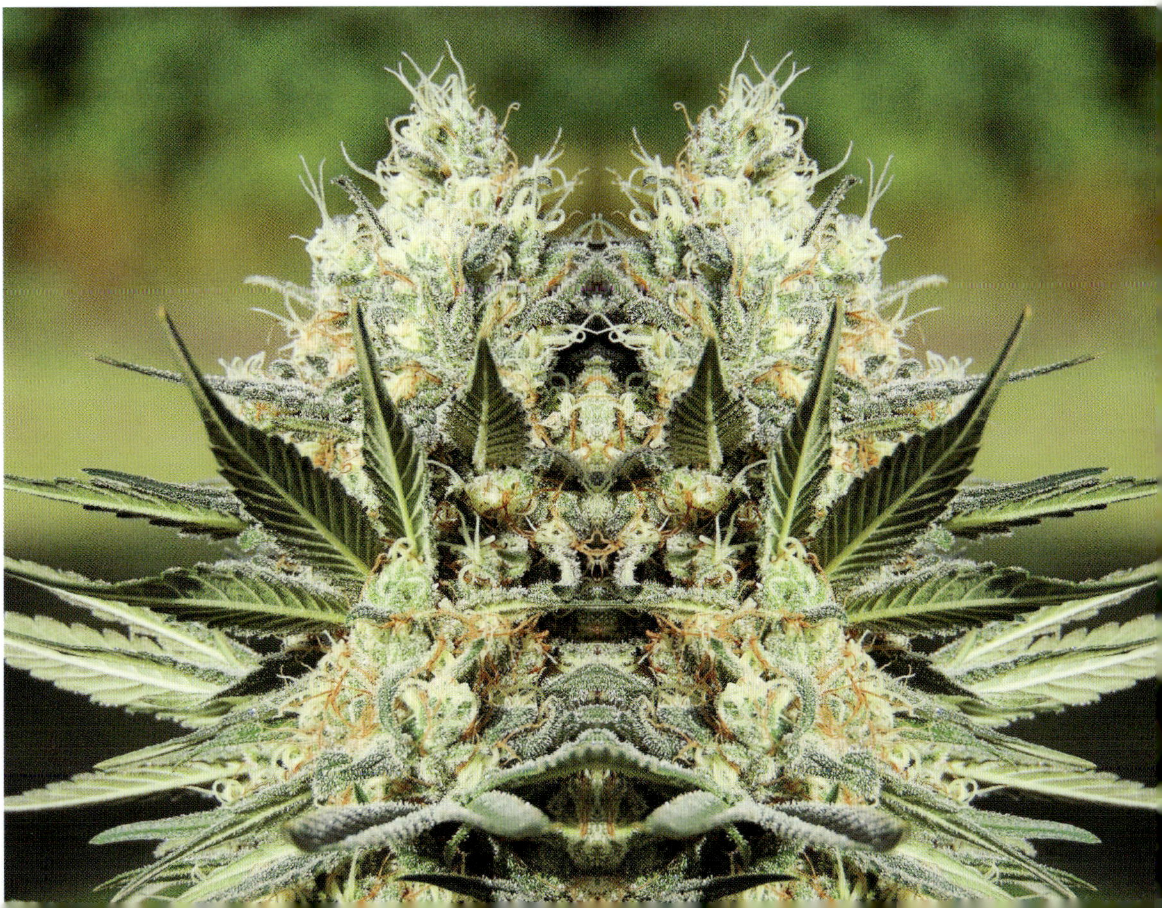

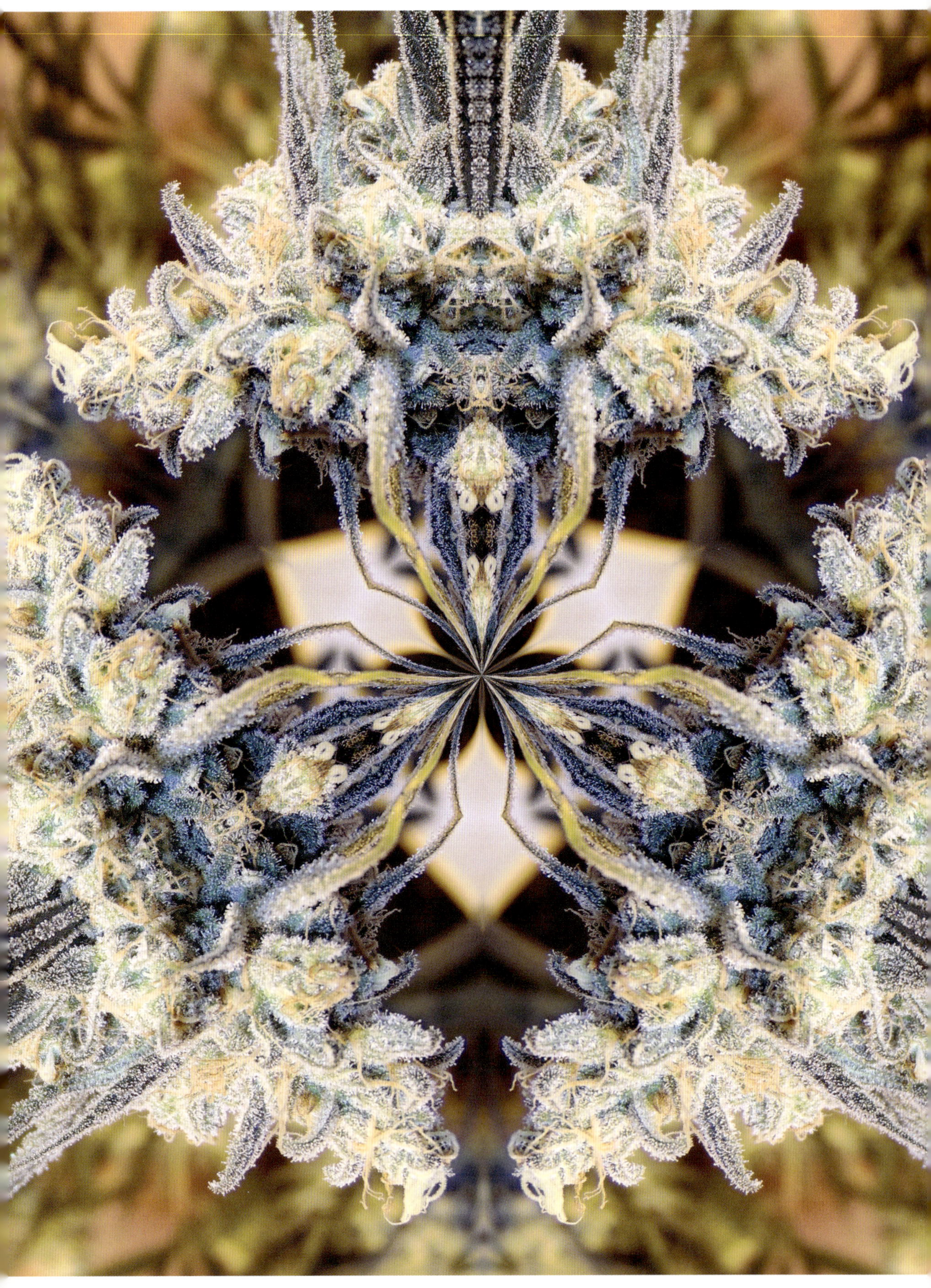

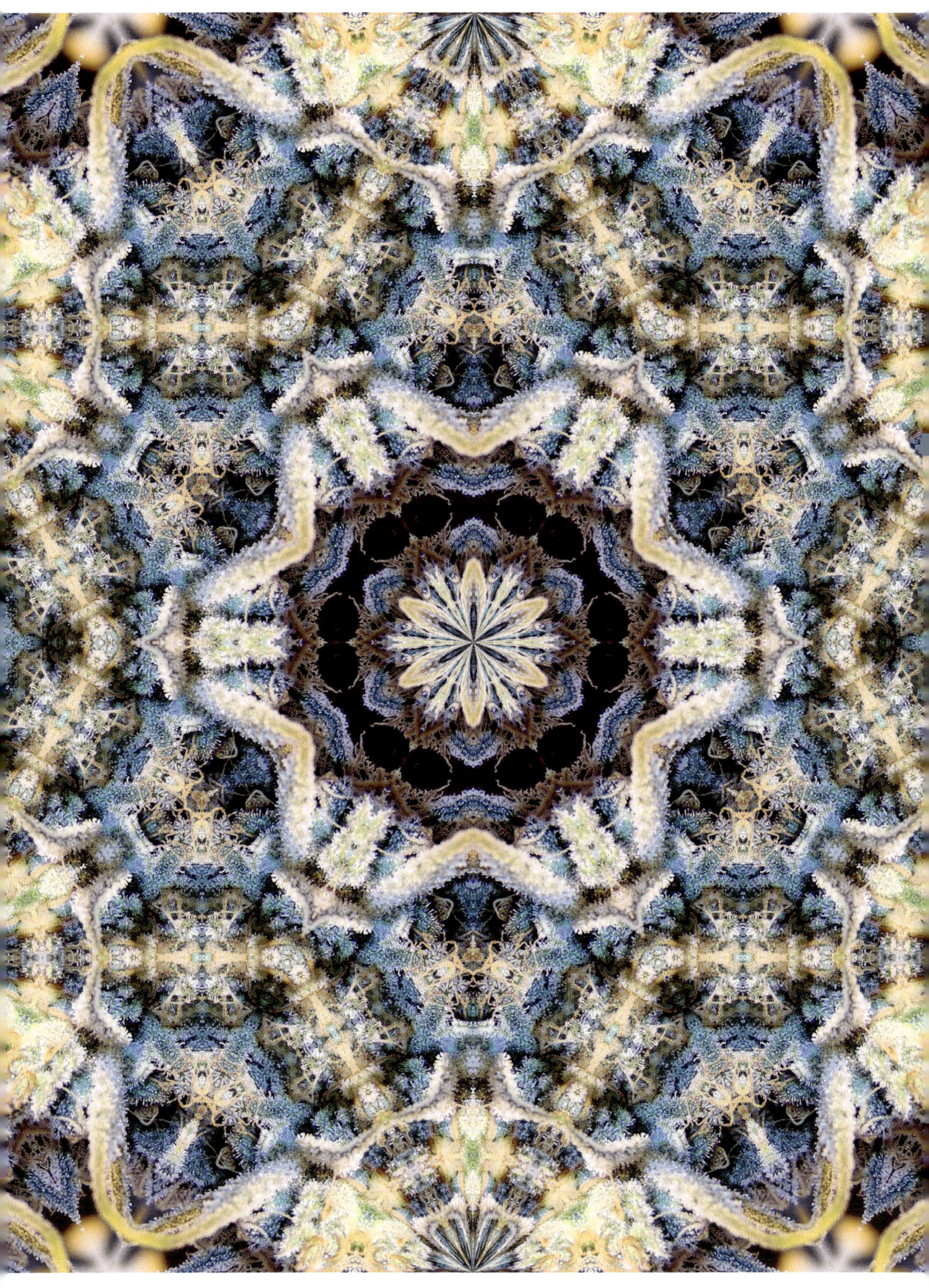

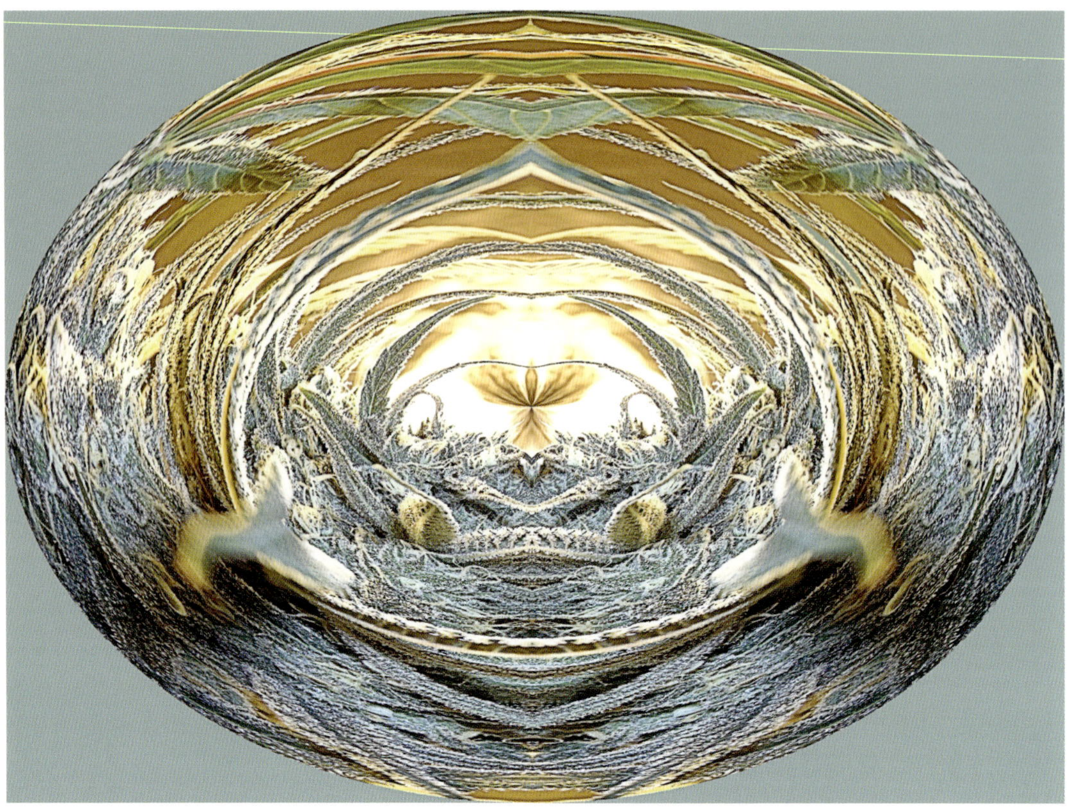

Spheroid

above—This spheroid lures you inward to the angelic figure in the center of the frame. Don't heed the call. You will get stuck in the resin and won't make it back out!

Ten Petals

following page—This ten-petal kaleidoscope eclipses the brown background. I see this image as a statement of unity. The cannabis sun contains beings holding hands as a gesture of love and compassion. They are celebrating the great gift of this flower. Humankind is together in peace and harmony once again.

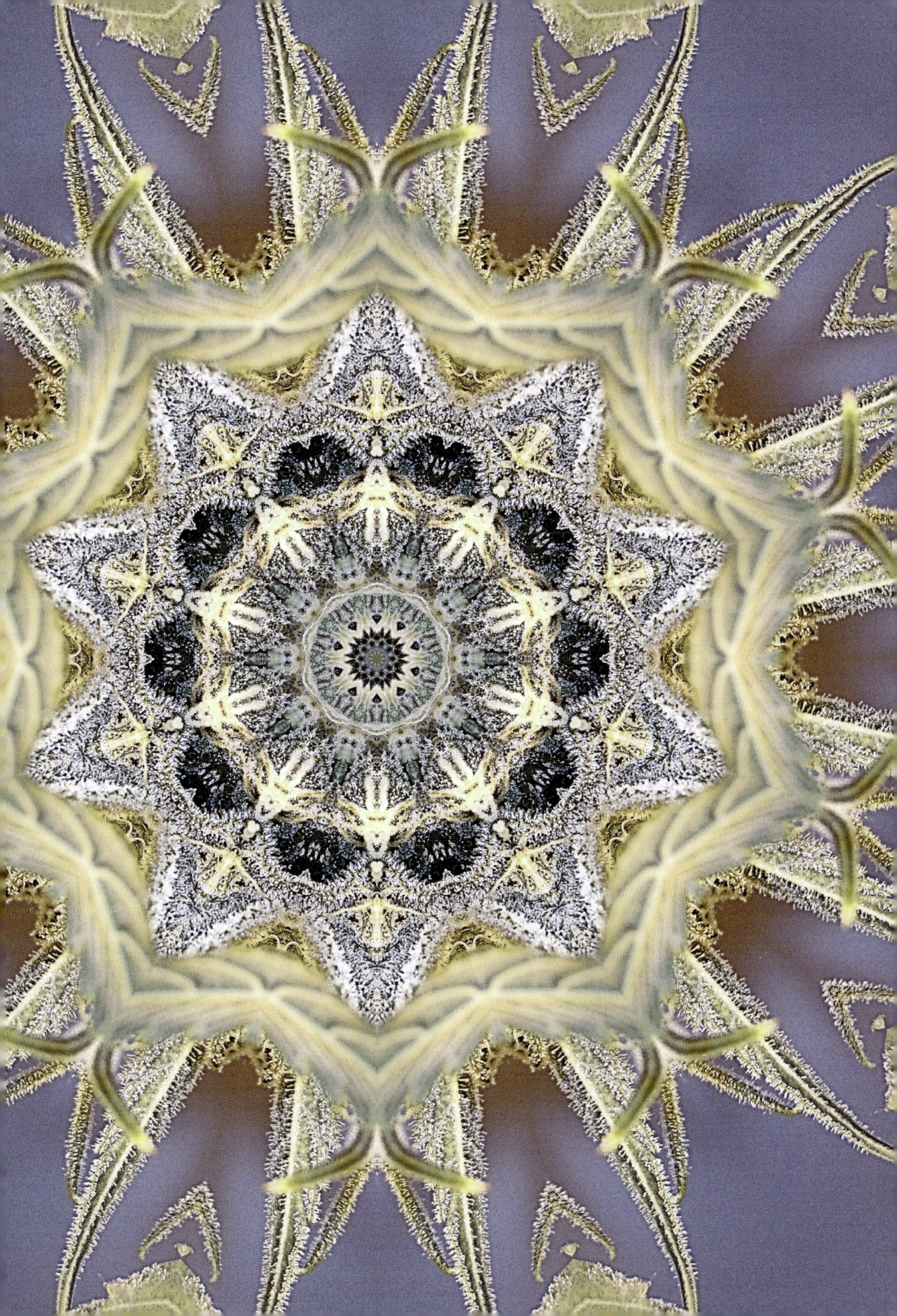

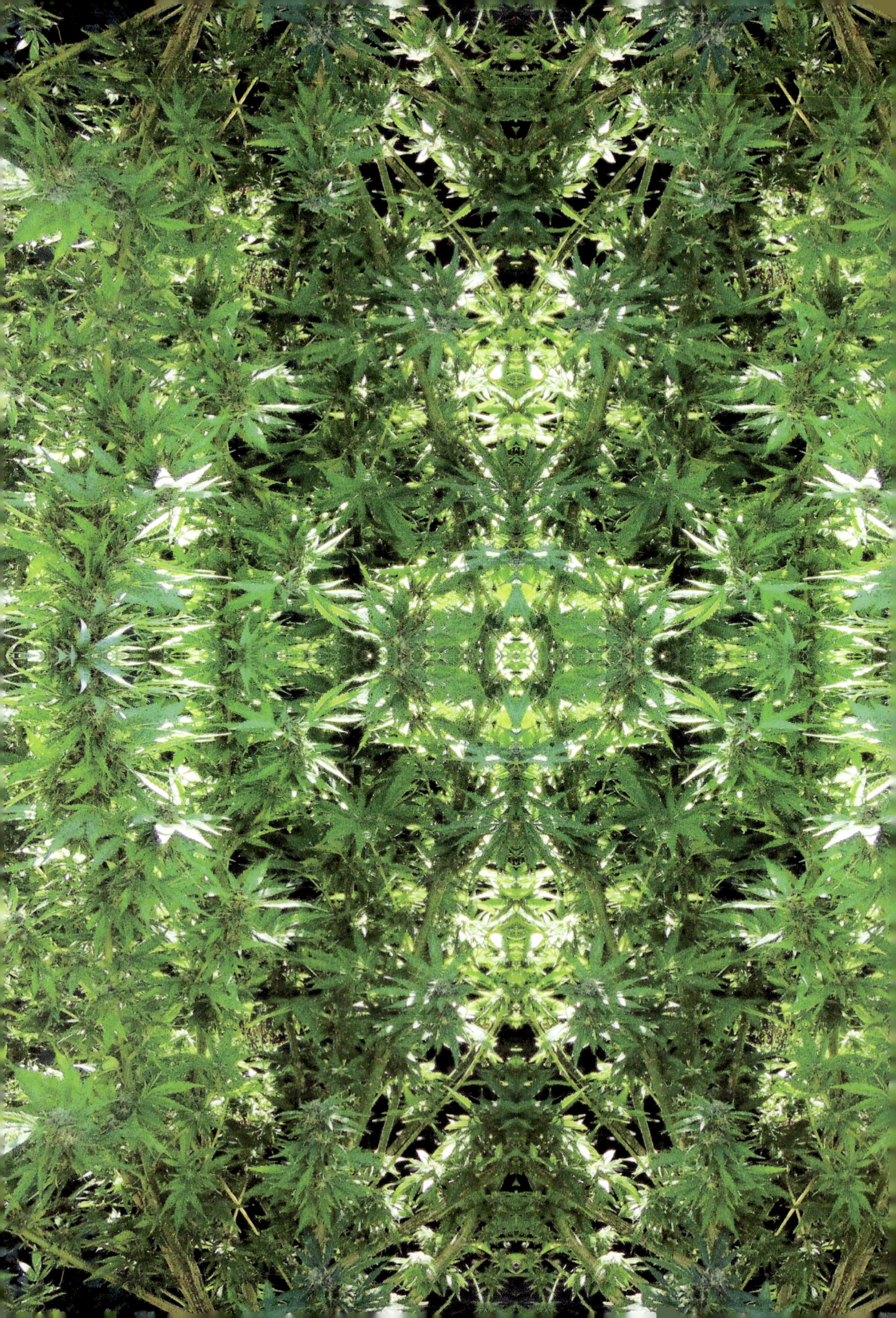

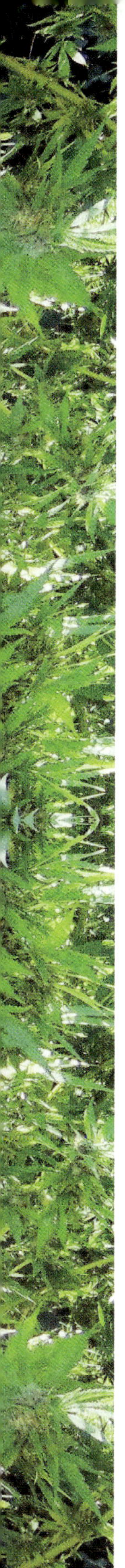

Entrapped

previous page—A dense bush has been mirrored, flipped, and mirrored again. The final image looks like another trap. It's for the DEA, though. The being's outer set of hands will grab the enemy and pull him in, while the inner hands will slap that agent silly until he vows to stop persecuting the plants. LMAO.

Wintry Mix

below—I'm always looking for nifty ideas for backgrounds, so I brought this Blue Dream babe outside to use the snow. The sun provided nice lighting on the buds and nice shadowing to the left.

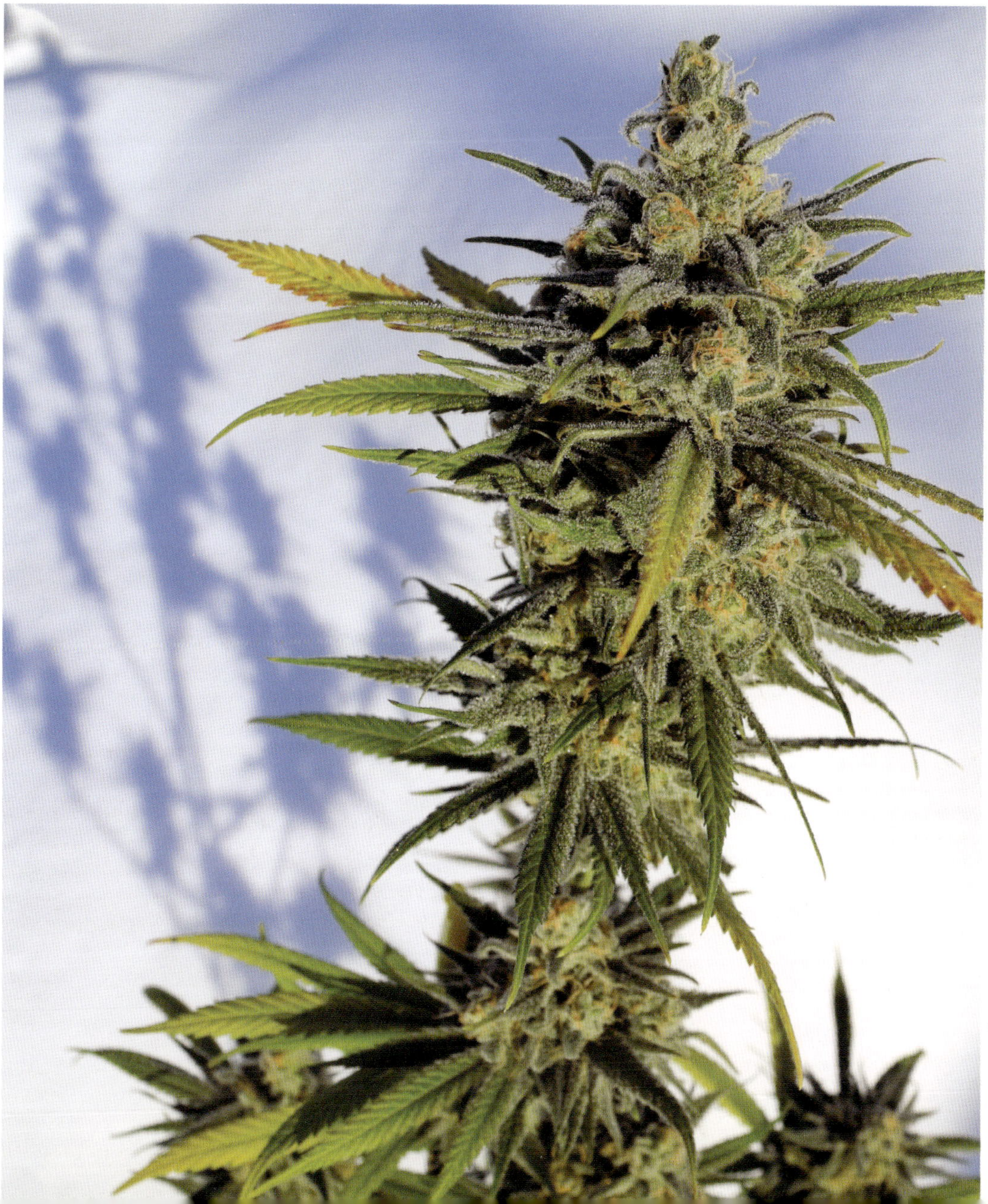

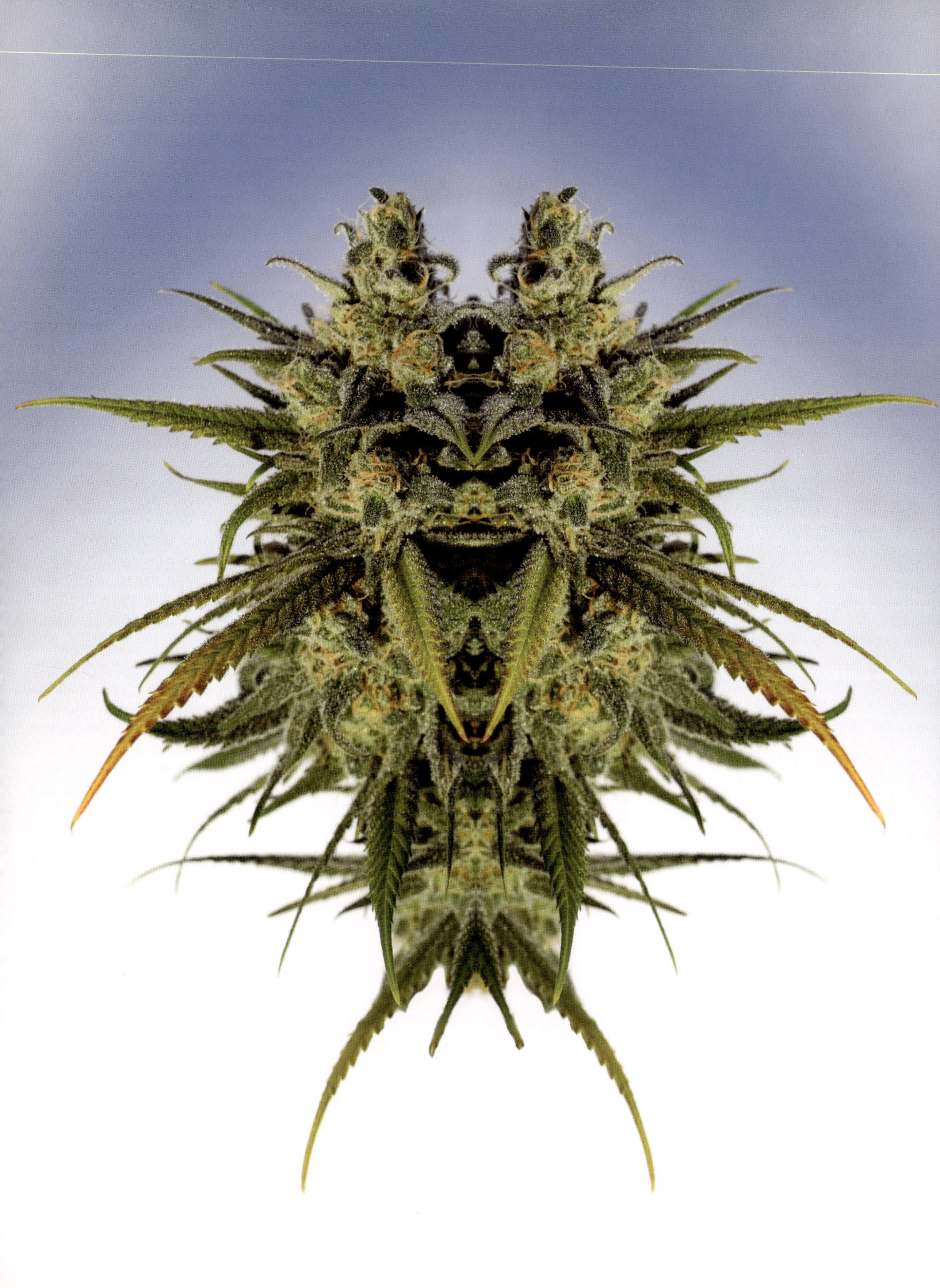

Archie

previous page—This one reminds me (and many people agree) of a friend named Archie. Rather than "goodbye," Archie says, "be happy." This image not only resembles his face in caricature, but the happy attitude he's adopted.

Another Look

below—The image on page 117 was used to create this one, as well. It is amazing to see what can be done with a less expensive camera and a decent, albeit aged, image-processing program.

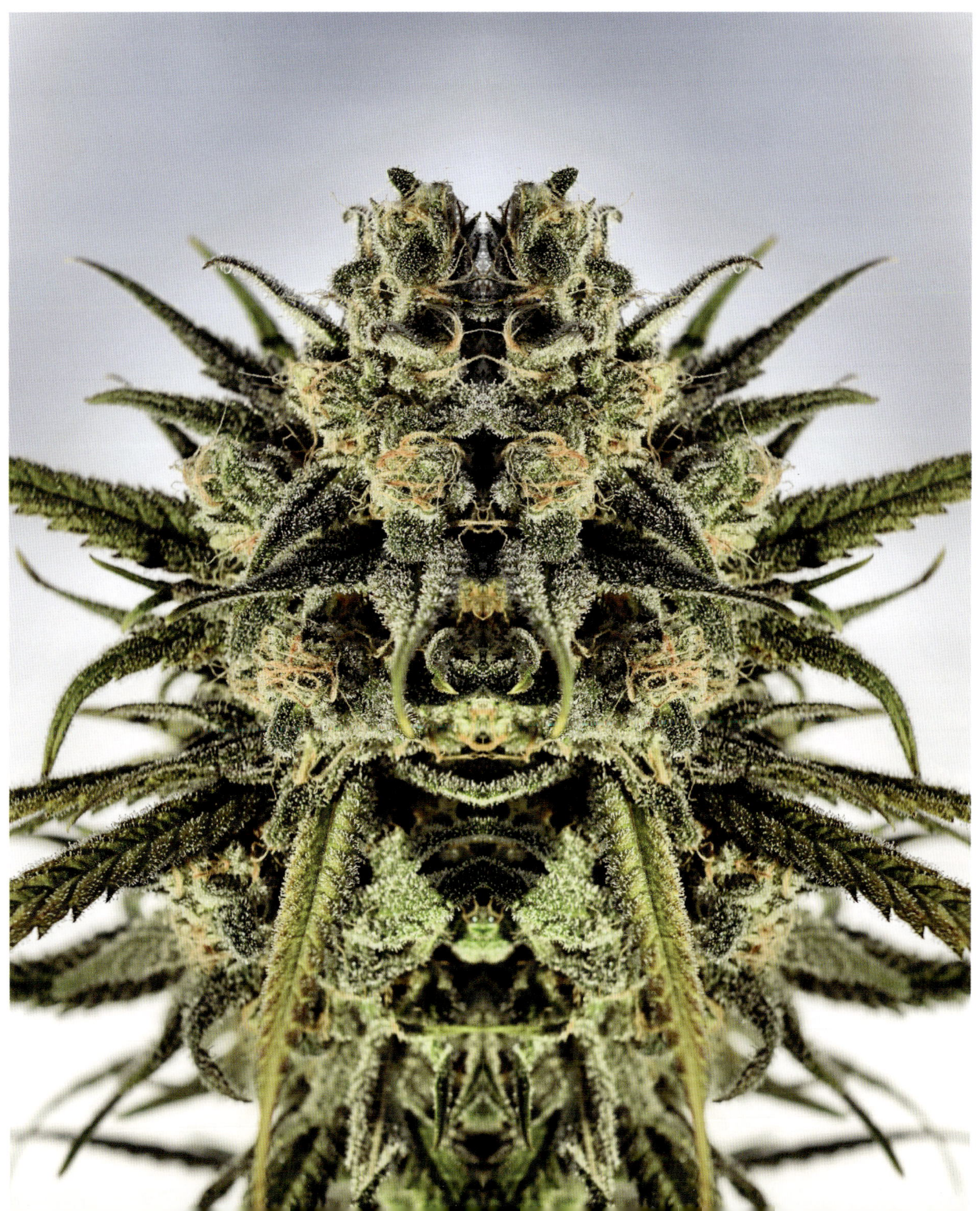

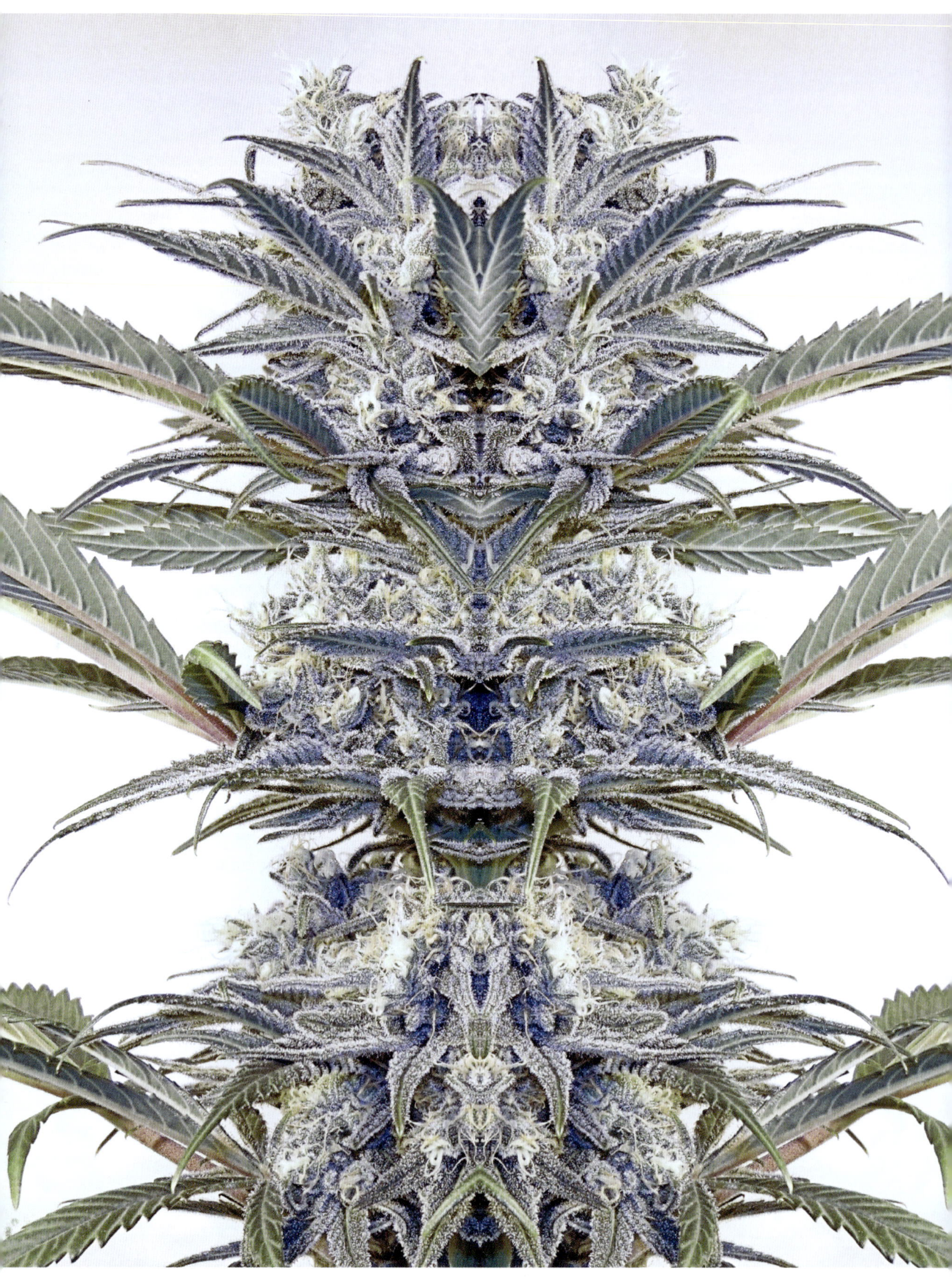

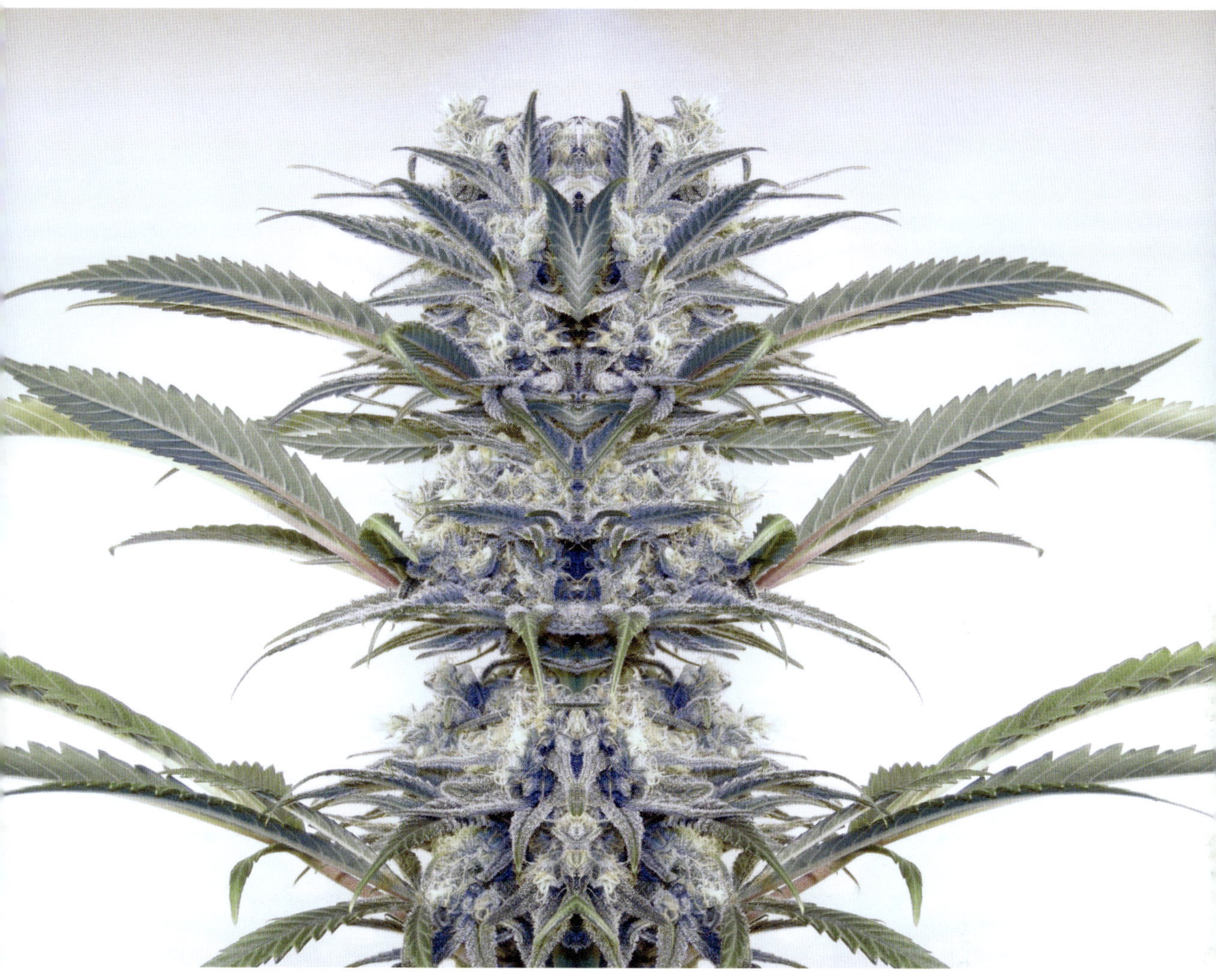

Fan Favorite

previous page—This image is a fan favorite. It's been called *The Totem* by many, so I've adopted that name for it. The blue color comes from a metal halide light, and it lends a unique look to the typically green buds.

Change in Format

above—Some images can be changed from a portrait format to a landscape. Doing this can allow me to create a harmonious group of framed photographs to be displayed on a wall. It's an approach that doesn't work with every image, though.

Grow Room

below—The original image of a slice of a grow room full of Blue Dream. Various stages are represented, with plants from one to six weeks of flowering.

following page—I mirrored the image below to get this totem. There are many faces in the center, with wall-to-wall green, healthy, organic goodness that will provide ample buds for months to come.

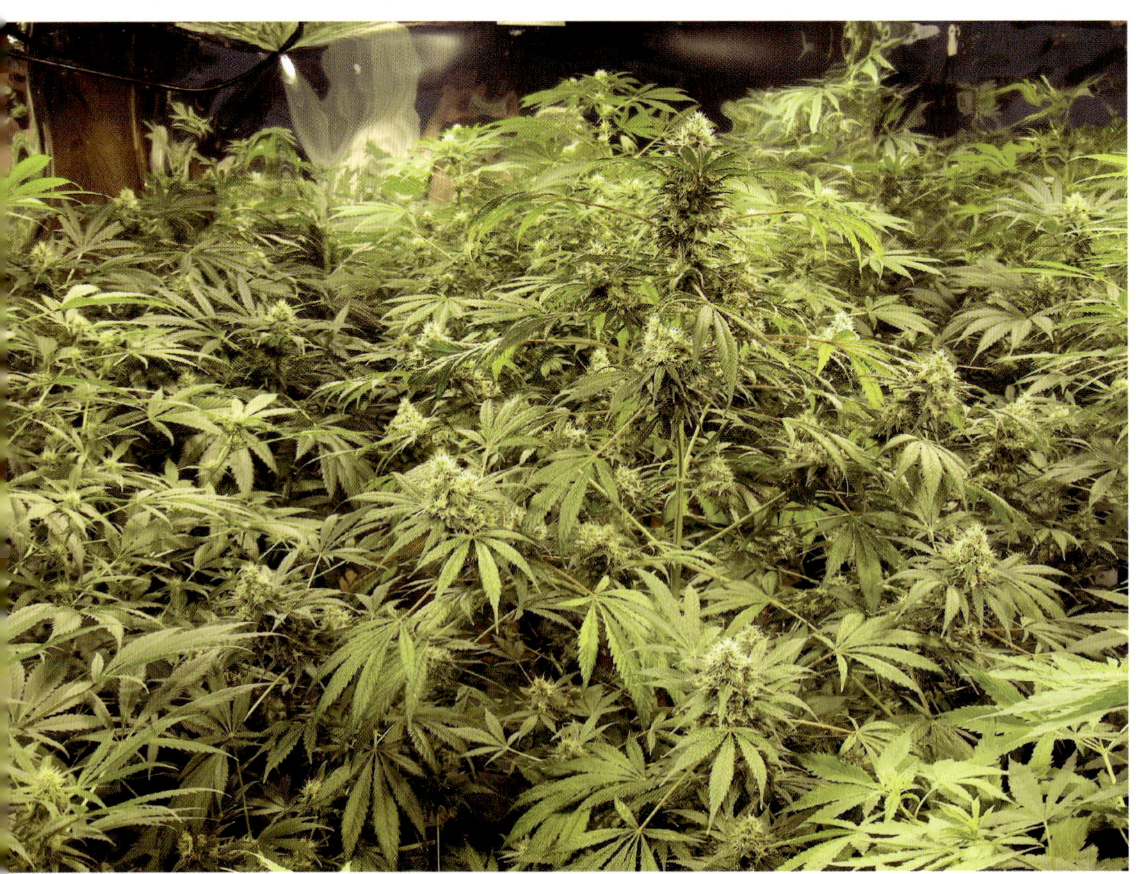

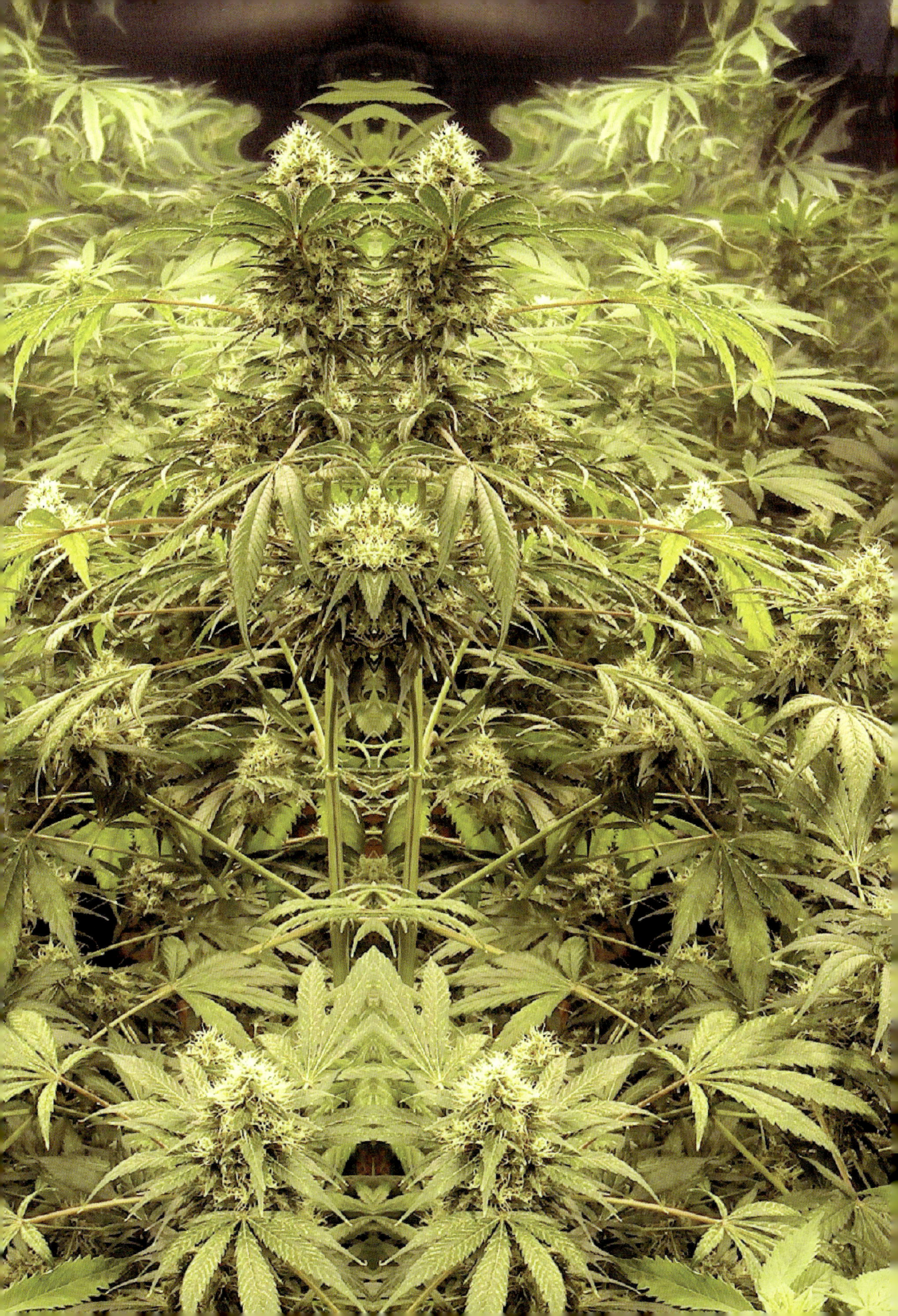

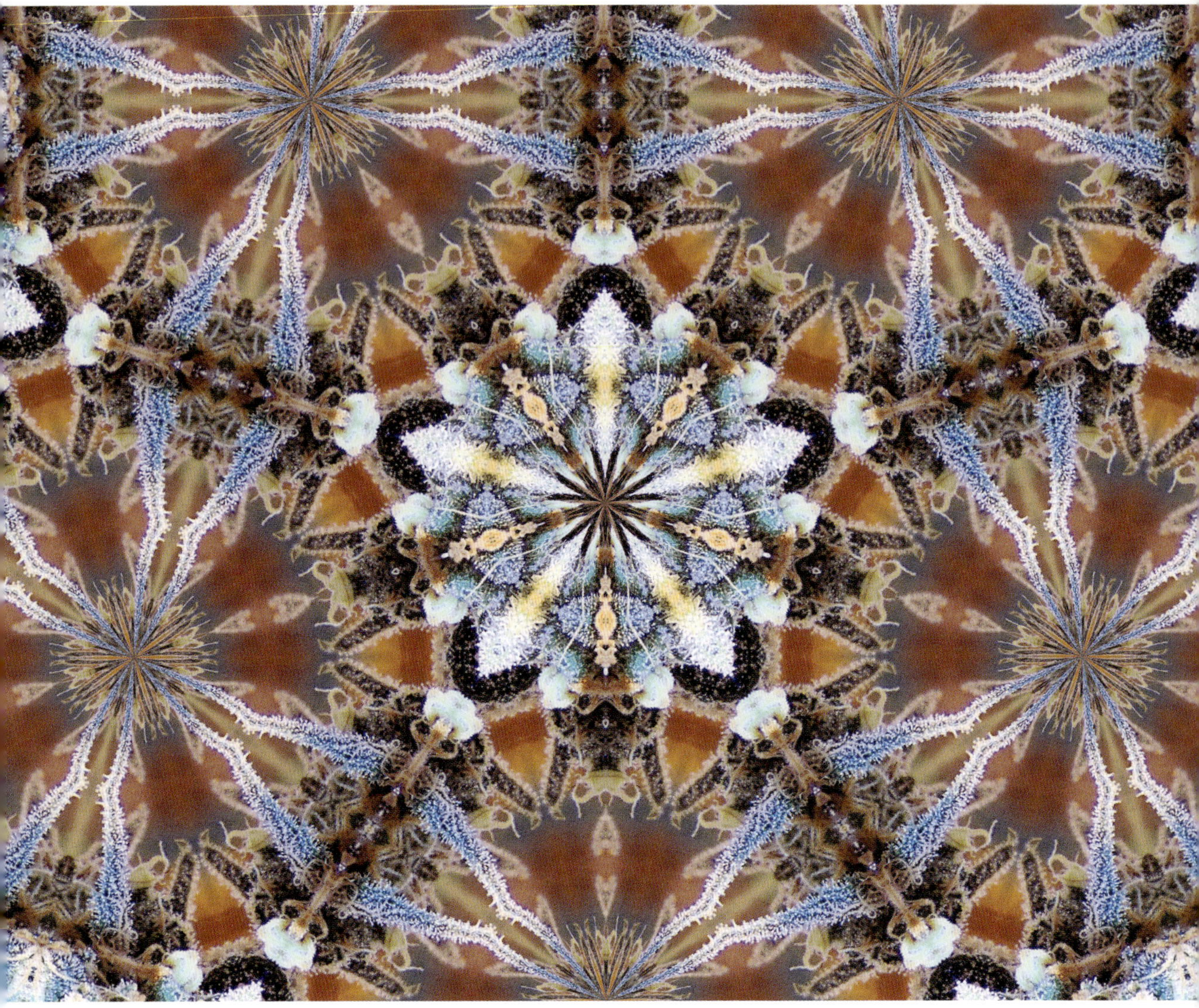

Five-Petal Mosaic

above—This beautiful five-petal mosaic that really impressed me. I hope you like it, too. It makes me think of a bedspread with this pattern on it.

Mary

following page—Meet Mary (not Brownie Mary!). She is 75 years old now and loves her cannabis—she eats it, drinks it, and smokes it. She's known in certain circles as "Granibus." Granibus? Yes! She has a t-shirt with the word on it, so it shall be! I've heard many times that she can out-smoke Willie Nelson, so I am issuing a challenge. If anyone can find Willie, email me at theartofcannabisbychris@gmail.com and let me know! Also, stop in and join my closed group on Facebook. Just search for The Art of Cannabis by Chris in the Facebook search bar.

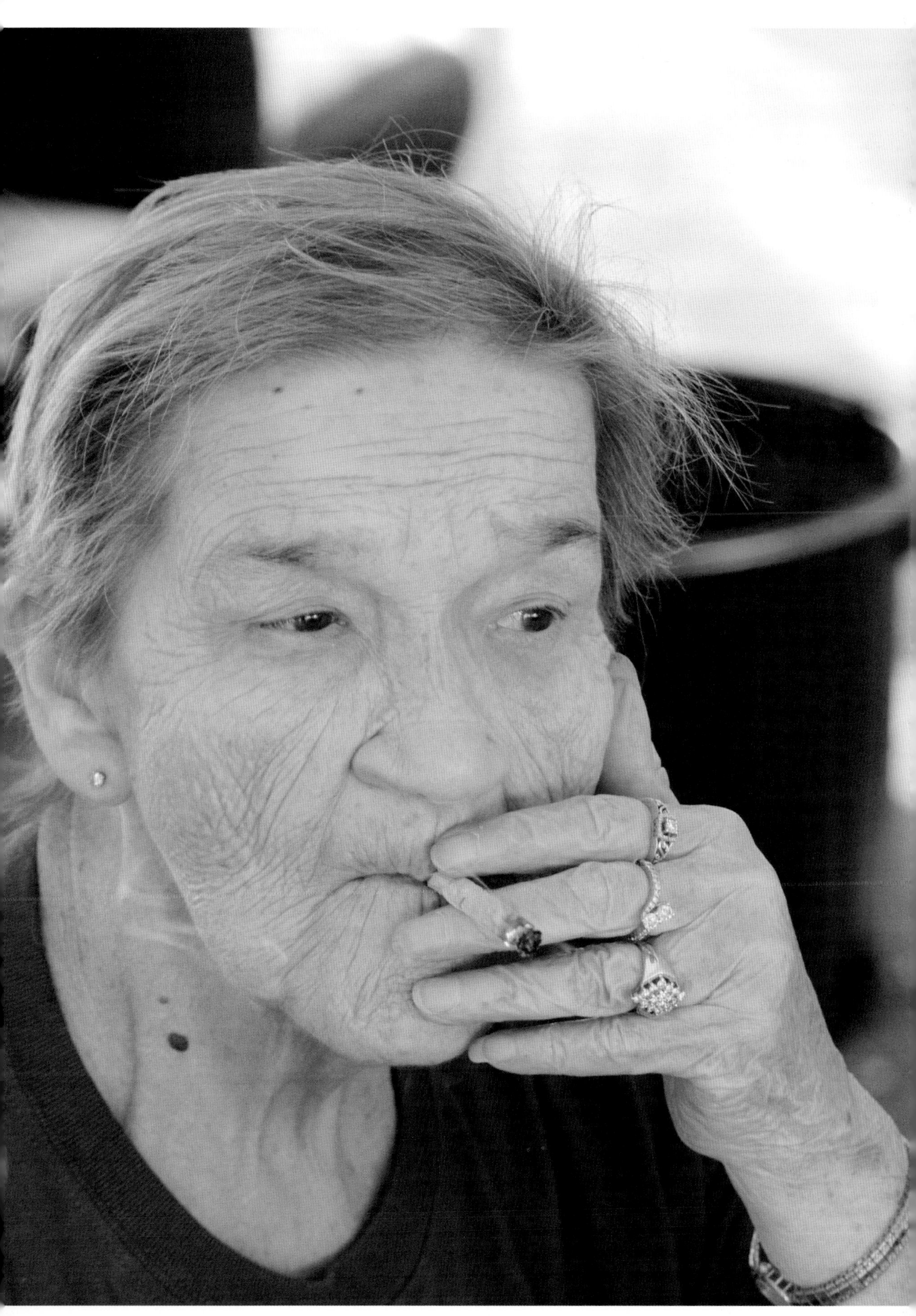

420

above—I know it's not a plant, but it's a real police car. I still revel in the fact that my wife saw this plate and told me about it. It took a little time for me to find the car, and I had to be stealthy to grab the image when the time was right. I had to clone out the Ford logo and and Michigan on the plate to use this image. I think it worked out pretty well.